Dr Roger Henderson

OVER-50s MEN'S HEALTH CHECK

PIATKUS

Copyright © 2004 by Roger Henderson

First published in 2004 by
Piatkus Books Ltd
5 Windmill Street
London W1T 2JA
e-mail: info@piatkus.co.uk

The moral right of the author has been asserted

*A catalogue record for this book is
available from the British Library*

ISBN 0 7499 2420 9

Edited by Krystyna Mayer
Text design by Paul Fielding

Set in Lapidary by Phoenix Photosetting, Chatham, Kent

Printed and bound in Great Britain by Mackays Ltd, Chatham, Kent

In memory of my father

CONTENTS

ACKNOWLEDGEMENTS

As with all my writing, my main thanks go to my long-suffering wife and children, who have become used to my frantic bursts of *Sturm und Drang* when deadlines loom near. In this regard, this book would never have been written without the understanding and patience of Judy Piatkus and Penny Philips, who tolerate my flexible definitions and musings as to what actually constitutes a final deadline with infinite patience. I must also thank Kim Dando for her secretarial skills, which truly came into their own at the eleventh hour.

I hope the end result has been worth it for all of these, and especially for that most endangered of species – the male.

Roger Henderson
March 2004

INTRODUCTION

'Be careful about reading health books. You may die of a misprint.'
— **Mark Twain**

As usual, Mark Twain was right on target here, and there is no question that in the 21st century we are as hooked on our health as we were in his day. But now, because of the overwhelming amount of information available to all at the click of a mouse, we are potentially better informed about our health than ever before. However, reading about health is one thing; understanding that information and acting on it when necessary is quite another. And when it comes to seeking advice about health problems, or even admitting we might have them in the first place, we men lag way behind women.

Let's face it: being a man is dangerous for your health. As a GP, whenever I sit down with a patient in my surgery and discuss health risk factors, there are three that are top of my list and which, unfortunately, I can do nothing about. The first is getting older. The second is a strong family history of certain conditions. The third is being male. When the good Lord was putting together his blueprints for men and women he must have got rather distracted when it came to men and wandered off leaving some loose ends that never really got tied up. For statistics now show that men die earlier than women in all age groups, are much more likely to take their own lives (up to eight times more in some age groups) and have a higher general level of illness from all cancers that are not gender-related.

It gets worse. In fact, in my idle moments I sometimes wonder whether being a man is not a disease in itself. (I suspect many long-suffering wives would agree.) When it comes to the state of men's health in the UK, there have been precious few encouraging signs over the past two or three decades. Men in low social classes still have a life expectancy at birth that is below the average male life expectancy of the early 1970s. Suicide rates for young men have more than doubled since 1971, as has the incidence of testicular cancer. Chronic liver disease increased fivefold between 1970 and 2000, while prostate cancer has increased by more than 130% since 1971. Male obesity has more than tripled over the same 30-odd years, and with it there has been an inexorable rise in levels of both Type 2 diabetes and heart disease.

Now, before the males among you who are reading this toddle off to the nearest pub in shock, not all is gloom and doom. As a result of the huge availability of health information I mentioned earlier, if some men are at last beginning to take an interest in their health, then their wives and partners certainly are too. It has been said that while being a man can seriously damage your health, having a female partner shortens the odds considerably. This benefit is often due to that woman frogmarching her unwilling husband or boyfriend down to the doctor to 'get sorted out'.

Despite this, men of all ages still remain seriously under-informed about the health issues that affect them, take unnecessary and excessive risks with their health and remain reluctant to seek advice from their doctor or health adviser, with only 1% being prepared to ask even their pharmacist about a health problem. (The next time you're in the chemist's, take a look not only at who is handing in prescriptions but also at how many of the over-the-counter products are exclusively or predominantly aimed at women.)

Why should this book on men's health – especially one aimed at those over 50 – be different from any that has gone before? Well, most books talk about men's health in general, whereas this one concentrates on the health issues that affect the largest group of men in the country – the over-50s. Late presentation of men with life-threatening but potentially treatable conditions, such as bowel and skin cancer, can be incredibly frustrating for doctors who know that earlier treatment would have increased the man's chances of survival.

Impotence is a problem which affects men over 50 in particular. More than half of all men between 40 and 70 have a problem with erectile dysfunction, yet most seek no help and nearly a third of those who have plucked up the courage to tell their doctor end up not accepting any treatment for it. Heart disease, diabetes, obesity, osteoporosis, depression and prostate cancer are some of the other issues that need to be addressed by this age group. And although everybody has to die of something, common illnesses are common, as I often tell my patients, and by concentrating on these you will greatly improve your chances of leading a healthier and longer life.

Prostate cancer is a good example. This is the second commonest cause of death in men and it is rare under the age of 50, but survival rates are greatly improved if it is both detected and treated early. However, many men do not attend their doctor until they begin to experience truly distressing symptoms, by which time the cancer has often spread outside the prostate gland. Many men are aware of potential problems with their prostate, but ask them where it is, or what symptoms they should be looking out for, and most will look at you blankly. A whole chapter of this book condenses all the crucial information about prostate cancer, its causes, symptoms and treatments, into accessible form, while the rest do the same with other conditions and problems that are of particular concern to men over 50.

I'm not a high-flying academic who scales ivory towers for a living. By contrast, as a family doctor I find myself dealing with the hard currency of men's health every single day. Just a few of the problems I see again and again are the man who has to get up three or four times a night to pass water, the obese man with chest pains, the previously happily married man who can't make love any more and the worried man who doesn't mention his health concerns for fear of what they may signify. Some do not require medication or treatment but a simple change in lifestyle or a natural treatment. Others will need substantial intervention. Whatever level of treatment is required, the key point remains the same – the more a man understands about his body and the sooner he seeks help for a problem (real or imagined), the better his prospects of remaining well. And, of course, the more often this happens, the quicker the great divide between men's and women's health will narrow.

Talking with my male patients, I'm sometimes reminded of the true story of a famous barrister who was renowned for his self-importance. A tetchy judge interrupted him in full flow and asked whether he felt he was wiser than his lordship and, if so, would he like to take over the case? Thinking fast, the barrister rose and said, 'Not wiser, my lord. Simply better informed.'

So, since we are looking at men's health as seen at the sharp end of general practice, here is a list of some salient and indeed salutary points:

- The average man can expect to be seriously or chronically ill for about 15 years of his life.
- Although the average male life expectancy at birth is some 75 years, if a man is partly skilled or unskilled this figure drops to below 70.
- Taken together, stroke and heart disease are the biggest single causes of male deaths in the UK, with the combined death rate from these two diseases being some 333 per 100,000 of the population.
- The second commonest cause of male deaths is cancer of all kinds, with a rate of 270 per 100,000 of the population.
- The number of new cases of prostate cancer diagnosed annually in the UK is expected to treble over the next 20 years from the current figure of 22,000 per year.
- The incidence of testicular cancer has doubled in the past 20 years and shows no sign of slowing.
- Not only are men as likely as women to be affected by depression, with one in five suffering from the illness at some point in their lives, but the suicide rate among men is increasing and among males of 15–24 has doubled over the past 25 years.
- At least 20% of men over 50 experience problems maintaining or achieving an erection and recent research suggests that a third of men of all ages say they climax too early.

- Forty-five per cent of men are overweight, nearly 20% are obese and just under 30% smoke, with the average male smoker consuming 111 cigarettes a week.
- Twenty-seven per cent of men drink more than the recommended limit of 21 units a week.

Quite a list, I think you will agree. Despite this, the evidence is that men – in the right environment – *will* ask questions about their health and are happy to use male-friendly health initiatives if provided. Unfortunately, such initiatives, for example clinics held in pubs and targeted well-man checks, are at present the exception rather than the rule. Increasing recognition by men and women of male health problems is probably being driven from the top down by dedicated health professionals rather than from the bottom up by the man in the street. This is not surprising, since women have lobbied far more successfully for changes in women's health-care than men appear willing to do for their sex. I suspect this is largely because men find it harder to discuss health issues and so are more reluctant to campaign as a group for political change in the way their health is dealt with.

This book is not intended to be a medical textbook and I hold my hand up to any charge that it is a little selective in the range of conditions it describes. However, not only does the small size of this book prevent me from writing about every male condition possible, but the ones I've focused on really are those I see most often, day in and day out.

Anyway, why are men so useless when it comes to looking after their health? What makes a man think nothing of lavishing hours of effort on his car, computer or work when he would baulk at spending a fraction of that time doing exercise or planning his diet? This is the big question and there are a number of familiar theories as to what the answer is. The obvious explanation is the macho myth that men can only be hard and indestructible. Never mind eating quiche, real men don't show a sensitive side and if they smoke and drink to excess then they've proved just how robust they are, and that's a man thing. Eight pints a night? Pah – you're just an amateur. This attitude makes it tricky for a man to admit to a doctor that he has any kind of health problem, so he will only turn up at the surgery when he is feeling so rough that even he knows something isn't quite right. Unfortunately, that's often too late.

Another cause is actually outside of men's control, so I can't blame them for this one. Men are designed to put on fat around their waists if they gain weight, but this 'beer belly' physique is worse for the heart than other body shapes, such as a big backside. Not only that, but our basic male sex hormone – testosterone – predisposes us to have more 'bad' cholesterol in our blood than women. I suppose it would help if men had babies, since then they would at least be aware of their reproductive cycle and as a result recognise the need to attend regular health checks. (Then again, if men did have babies, they'd either pay someone else to have one for them or design a machine that did it on their behalf.)

We remain uneducated in so many areas of health. But I hope this book will, at the very least, allow men (and their partners) to understand the danger areas that being male can lead them into and – more importantly – the simple ways to avoid going down those particular paths. One of my favourite quotes concerning a man and his health comes from George Foreman, the champion heavyweight boxer who regained his title when he was nearer 50 than 40 but who is now perhaps better known for promoting his low-fat grilling machine. 'I have the body of a man half my age,' he said. 'Unfortunately, he's in terrible shape.' The trouble is, millions of men in this country could truthfully say the same thing, but if this book saves just one of them from a premature death, then it will have been a worthwhile venture. Above all, remember that, for the vast majority of men, good health comes down to one overriding thing – common sense. Follow this simple advice and you're well on your way to taking care of yourself.

Good health.

1
HEART DISEASE

'Do excuse me, but I'm having a coronary thrombosis.'
– **Montgomery of Alamein,** *while suffering a heart
attack in the House of Lords*

Heart disease is one of those terms that everybody knows
and talks about. But, because it covers many conditions, if
you are not careful it can become more and more complicated the more you look at it. This is a shame as the heart is
basically a pump (a very complex one, but still a pump) and
so probably the best way to think about it is in terms of
plumbing.

When I'm talking to my patients over 50, though, what I
really mean is coronary heart disease, or ischaemic heart
disease. This occurs when there is a progressive silting up of
the fine blood vessels around the heart, usually by fat and
other debris, and this takes place over many years. Silting up
of the blood vessels narrows the arteries so that they are
increasingly less able to carry blood and oxygen to the
muscles of the heart, with the result that the heart has to
pump harder to send blood around the body. This can cause
the heart to fail progressively in its job as a pump and leads
to symptoms such as pain in and around the chest, breathlessness and heart failure. The eventual result is a heart
attack, of which there are almost 300,000 in the UK every

year, while a further two million people experience chest pain owing to heart disease.

Heart disease is the greatest cause of ill health and death in the Western world and a major player in the health of its over-50s. The UK has a poor record for heart disease, currently lying eighth, out of 21 countries from four continents, in the World Health Organisation's heart-disease monitoring table. I'm no great fan of statistics but I readily accept that 41% of all deaths in this country are from heart-related conditions.

So, a big problem – right? Right. Therefore if we understand what causes heart disease we can try to do something about it and keep ourselves living longer and healthier. The heart beats some 2.5 billion times in a 70–80 year lifespan, so it makes sense if our arteries remain clear and unblocked so that the blood can whiz round them freely. They also need to have a degree of elasticity so that they can widen to send more blood to our muscles during exercise. Just as our domestic water pipes fur up with limescale, so calcium and cholesterol harden into a material known as plaque, which, once present, is very hard to remove. I've seen deposits of plaque at post-mortem which are as hard as brick. Let's take a look at some of the risk factors that predispose us to both plaque and heart disease in general.

RISK FACTORS

As I often say to my male patients, there are three factors in heart disease over which we have no control. The first is getting old. Sorry about that, but there we are. The second is being a man. Unfortunately, men are at considerably greater risk of developing heart disease then women. While this condition accounts for nearly a third of all male deaths in the UK, the corresponding figure for female deaths is 22%. Up to the age of 50, deaths from heart disease are six or seven times higher in men than in women, although women catch up after the menopause and by the age of 75 there is virtually no difference in risk.

The third factor we have no say over is our genes. As someone with, shall we say, an interesting family history of heart disease, this is a subject of some importance to me because in such cases it can occur even though there are no other obvious significant risk factors. However, for many people, family-linked problems of heart disease such as high cholesterol, high blood pressure and diabetes are well-recognised precipitating factors. In real terms this means that the majority of men start on a level playing field and either develop new risk factors or choose not to do anything about the ones already in existence.

Let's now look at the other risk factors commonly involved in heart disease in men over 50.

● **High blood pressure (hypertension).** One in five of the UK population is likely to develop high blood pressure, but in the majority of cases there is no obvious cause – it simply happens. This is known as essential or primary hypertension. Blood pressure with an obvious cause is known as secondary hypertension and here it is often kidney problems or other biochemical abnormalities that contribute to the condition. The main effect of both kinds of hypertension is not only sometimes to accelerate the build-up of plaque in the blood vessels but also to increase general wear and tear on the arteries of the heart and body.

● **High cholesterol.** Doctors seem to like cholesterol because it comes in nice round figures, it is an undisputed risk in heart disease and it can be treated by simple lifestyle changes or, failing this, simple drug treatment. Over recent years what counts as a level of cholesterol needing attention has become something of a moveable feast. I remember as a medical student doctors quite happily accepting amounts of cholesterol in their patients which now make my eyes water when I think about it.

Cholesterol is a fairly innocuous fatty substance produced by the liver on a steady basis and found in our circulation and around our nerves. It is not the evil entity that we often accuse it of being but is a prerequisite of the bile acids we need to help digest food. The science here is basically that it is carried around the blood by substances called lipo-proteins. The two important types of these that doctors get excited about are high-density lipoproteins (HDL or 'good' cholesterol) and low-density lipoproteins (LDL or 'bad' cholesterol).

About three-quarters of our cholesterol is made from our own body, with the rest coming from our diet. It is our liver that pumps out LDL to take cholesterol around the body, but on its journey some of this LDL can leave deposits of cholesterol along the walls of our blood vessels. Not good. It is the job of HDL to try to pick up some of these deposits and take them back to the liver for recycling and disposal. (In my idler moments I've imagined that HDL looks like dustmen sweeping up as they go but still leaving occasional rubbish behind.) If you're over 50, knowing what your cholesterol level is and taking action to bring it down if it is high is one of the best things you can do for your heart.

● **Obesity.** It is not often I use the word epidemic but I think that when we are talking about obesity it is completely justified. In the next decade we are heading for an epidemic of obesity throughout the Western world the like of which we have never seen. This not only applies to men over 50 but even to teenagers and children of both sexes as young as nine or ten. The two driving forces for this explosion in obesity are an increasingly sedentary lifestyle and consumption of ever-bigger portions of calorie-rich food and snacks.

When we pile on weight as body fat, this not only tends to increase our blood pressure but also pushes up our levels of LDL cholesterol and makes us more prone to conditions such as diabetes, which is itself a risk factor for heart disease. Being fat is bad for you, but the distribution of that fat also influences our risk of heart problems. In a nutshell, people with a big belly are at greatest risk of all as they often have very low levels of HDL cholesterol, and it is in this part of the body that most men find they put their weight on as they grow older.

● **Diabetes.** This is a disorder of carbohydrate metabolism; in other words, people with diabetes are less able to regulate their blood sugar levels than people who don't have the disease. All diabetics have an increased risk of heart disease and in the over-50s the mortality rate from this cause is twice that of people without diabetes. This increased risk is mainly due to the effect of diabetes on the very fine circulation in the body as it makes it more prone to sludging up and blocking. Diabetes and the increase in obesity in our society seem to be running in parallel, and indeed one of the first-line treatments of diabetes is simple weight loss.

We've considered individually four of the very big hitters

that can cause heart disease in people of all ages, but we should think of this problem as being due to a number of risk factors rather than just one. I often say that a heart attack is the end result of a jigsaw that is gradually put together over many years, and when the final piece is slotted into place the heart attack or episode of angina occurs. From where I sit it's clear that there are also other crucial factors in the development of heart disease.

● **Smoking.** King of the hill, top of the heap, number-one enemy, whatever you want to call it, this is the big one. I'm no health fascist, but if there was one thing in the world I would do with a magic wand it would be to stop people smoking. Even the nicotine from one cigarette is enough to narrow a small artery, and continuing to smoke into middle age doubles the risk of heart disease. Smoking has its own chapter later in the book, but it's worth saying here too that when you inhale from a cigarette, damaging molecules called free radicals are released into the body and these dramatically speed up plaque formation in the arteries as well as putting such delights as cyanide and arsenic into the bloodstream. I sometimes muse on the irony that some people who exercise regularly and are fastidious in checking their cholesterol levels will happily get through 10 or 20 cigarettes a day and convince themselves that these careful measures are offsetting any harm done by smoking.

● **Alcohol.** In excess – and this is the key phrase – alcohol not only increases your blood pressure but can push up your blood fat levels as well. It is interesting that both heavy drinkers and teetotallers appear to have a slightly raised risk of heart disease compared with moderate drinkers. I like to think I'm one of these, although you may remember that one definition of an alcoholic is someone who drinks more than their doctor. Men should aim to drink less than 21 units of alcohol a week, where one unit is half a pint of average-strength beer, a pub measure of spirits or a standard glass of wine. If the world of wine made a list of issues where clear thinking gets bogged down in a morass of half-truths, the question of wine's health benefits would surely be near the top. Is wine healthy at all? How much is too much? Is it only red wine we should be talking about, and, if so, is a '61 Petrus better for you than a '99 Chilean Cabernet?

Before attempting to answer these questions, let's go back to 1991 and the American TV programme *60 Minutes*. Hardly anyone remembers this show but it was an important event in medical terms as it was the first time that people heard those two sexy words 'French paradox' explained and discussed. The programme looked at the lower incidence of heart disease in the French compared with Americans and suggested that this was entirely due to wine's protective benefit to the heart and circulation. Four years later the same programme revisited this question, presenting new evidence from Denmark, where wine appeared to have greater health benefits than other alcoholic drinks, such as beer and spirits. Since 1995 our understanding of the possible reasons why wine, and red in particular, may be good for us has improved dramatically and there are certain general points that most people now accept.

The first is that the health benefits of wine are highly likely to be derived from phenolic compounds, which are found in high concentrations in grape skins, seeds and stems. These compounds, more often referred to as antioxidants, appear to be beneficial in two ways. Firstly, they help prevent 'bad' cholesterol (LDL) from being laid down as unhealthy plaque that can clog up and block blood vessels. Secondly, they reduce the chances of blood clots developing in the body by slightly thinning the blood, especially if wine is drunk during a meal. In addition to these circulatory benefits, there is now also evidence to suggest that antioxidants help in the fight against free radicals – naturally occurring and harmful products in our body cells that have been implicated in the development of certain cancers and Alzheimer's disease.

If antioxidants are beneficial, are all wines equally 'healthy'? Well, no. Red wines in general contain more antioxidants than white wine (and in this respect top the league table of all alcoholic drinks), but even among red wines there are premier-league vineyards that we should look for. Red burgundy, Merlot, Pinot Noir and, king of them all, Chilean Cabernet seem to have the highest levels of the antioxidants resveratrol and flavonol. Chilean grapes are normally harvested later than those in less warm climates and this allows a greater concentration of antioxidants to develop in the grapes before they are picked. The wine-pressing techniques used to make South American wines are also more vigorous than those of other countries, with the result that the small grapes and their seeds produce a higher concentration of these beneficial chemicals. Very important to this question of wine's health benefits is the wine-making process itself, which uses all parts of the grape and is essentially an anaerobic (without oxygen) activity. By contrast, it is believed that the prolonged exposure to air that characterises open fermentation may destroy naturally occurring antioxidants. This would explain why grape juice, for example, does not appear to have the same beneficial effect as red wine.

The next question is, when should we be drinking? Almost certainly the answer is, with food. It is this element that may well explain the French paradox since, despite their fat-rich diet, the French are four times less likely to die from heart disease than the average person in the UK. As most wine is drunk with food in France, Spain and Italy – all countries with lower levels of heart disease and higher wine consumption than the UK – it may be this pattern of drinking, rather than the binge drinking so often seen here, that makes the important difference. There is, however, an important caveat. It is only in the past two decades or so that the French and British have been consuming equivalent quantities of cholesterol, and it is the French who have been doing the catching up. If the incidence of heart disease in France starts to rise over the next decade, the French paradox may be turned on its head, although most experts believe this is unlikely.

So, you are looking expectantly at your chosen wine while savouring the aroma of your favourite meal. Unfortunately for lovers of wine, more is not better, and doubling your intake will not double the health benefits. There is a very fine line between healthy drinking and drinking more than is good for you, with both teetotallers and drinkers of more than four or five units a day having an increased risk of heart disease compared with moderate drinkers. This protective effect increases with age, with the most marked benefits becoming apparent in those over 60. It must be stressed, though, that wine is not the panacea for all infirmities. Louis Pasteur may have said, 'Wine is the most healthful and hygienic of beverages', but by itself it can't fight off the effects of smoking, obesity, raised blood pressure and lack of exercise. However, as part of a generally healthy lifestyle, it is quite possibly the most palatable medicine ever invented.

● **Stress.** Does stress cause heart attacks? The answer is almost certainly no, but my take on this is that a stressful lifestyle often leads to riskier behaviour, such as an increase in smoking and drinking. Also, over a long time stress may elevate our blood pressure. In connection with this it was believed at one time that there were two distinct personalities and that these could influence the risk of heart disease. The Type A personality was a highly strung, rather irritable and impatient person who ate and talked rapidly and tended to be very achievement-orientated. The Type B personality was calmer, slightly less ambitious and generally took life at a more relaxed pace. This personality was not bothered by queues or delays, and less prone to frustration or anger. Most authorities now recognise that these are rather imprecise definitions and that the majority of us veer between one and the other most of the time. However, there is wide agreement that it is far better to be relaxed most of the time than stressed, and this is something that can be achieved with practice. There are countless books, along with recorded material in all formats and advice on the internet, that teach effective relaxation techniques.

● **Sedentary lifestyle.** In the main we all take far less exercise than we did a hundred years ago. We leave our house with all mod cons to go to work in our car, sit at a desk all day, then come back home in the car to sit on the sofa eating our calorie-rich TV dinner. OK, this may be slightly pushing the point but a lot of people do all this and take no or little exercise. You do not have to be an Olympian to benefit from exercise as it takes only 20–30 minutes of moderate activity three times a week – for example, walking briskly, swimming or cycling – to achieve appreciable health benefits. The real problem with a sedentary lifestyle is that it predisposes to obesity, which in turn gives rise to other risk factors.

ANGINA AND HEART ATTACK

We've mentioned angina and heart attack as common effects of heart disease. Let's look at these in more detail.

Angina is a transient pain, usually in the middle of the chest but often radiating into the arms, neck or jaw. It occurs when an area of the heart muscle does not get enough of the oxygen it requires and goes into cramp. Although it is unusual for a simple angina attack to progress into a full-blown heart attack, if you are a man over 50 it is certainly an indicator that you are at risk of having one later in life. For this reason it must always be taken seriously. The symptoms vary from individual to individual but most sufferers describe a sudden onset of central chest pain, often after exertion such as mowing the lawn or having sex, and there may be aching in both arms but more especially on the left side. Rest tends to bring a quick reduction in the pain, but there may be a general feeling of breathlessness and men have told me that they have felt as though they were suffocating during an attack. Treatment with GTN (glyceryl trinitrate), in the form of a spray used under the tongue or tablets, tends to relieve the pain very quickly.

A heart attack, whether referred to as a coronary throm-bosis, myocardial infarction or major ischaemic episode, is still exactly that – an attack on the heart muscle itself.

Instead of this simply going into cramp, as with angina, during a heart attack part of the muscle actually dies because its blood supply is completely blocked off. At least a third of all men who die prematurely do so from a heart attack. The most typical symptom is a sudden severe crushing pain in the middle of the chest, sometimes accompanied by sweating, nausea and vomiting and occasionally burping or belching. There is often breathlessness and a feeling of anxiety, and in many cases the pain spreads into the neck and jaw and down into the arms, although this is highly variable. The heart may feel like it is beating a rapid but irregular tattoo and in a major attack it can stop altogether.

New techniques to determine whether someone has suffered an episode of angina or a heart attack continue to be introduced but old-fashioned ones are still in use. These include an electrocardiogram (ECG), in which electrodes are painlessly attached to the chest, arms and legs to record the electrical activity of the heart and the heartbeat. This allows doctors to see if any changes in the heart muscle have occurred and it highlights areas of the heart that are not functioning or have been deprived of oxygen. A true heart attack produces a characteristic tracing on an ECG, but if the results appear normal or the changes are very mild, then doctors may use relatively new and very sensitive blood tests to check if there has been recent damage to heart muscle cells.

A progression from a simple ECG is an exercise stress test, where an ECG is carried out while the patient is exercising, usually on a treadmill. This is a very good preventive tool as it allows doctors to evaluate whether the patient has what is called significant angina and how likely it is that this will lead to a heart attack.

Imaging tests can also be used. These include echocardiograms, which are ultrasound tests that display an image of the heart transmitted from a simple ultrasound transducer placed on the chest (similar to those used on pregnant women). They are very good at showing up any problems with heart valves or areas of heart muscle that have been significantly damaged. Another way of producing a good image of the heart is an MRI scan, which produces a three-dimensional picture of the heart. However, current pressures on the NHS's scanning machines do not allow these to be routinely used for patients with angina.

Doctors may move on to more invasive tests which, although they carry a slightly greater risk of harm than the previously mentioned tests, are very efficient for doctor and patient alike. The commonest of these is a coronary angiogram, in which a small catheter is inserted into an artery (usually in the groin or arm) and a radio-opaque dye is injected into the body through this. This allows a map of the heart and blood vessels to be recorded and subsequently analysed to see if there are any blockages as the dye-highlighted blood flows through the heart. At the same time that this is being done, a technique known as cardiac catheterisation may also occur; this looks at the blood flow through the heart and how effectively the heart is pumping.

After going through some or all of these tests, most patients can be accurately diagnosed and treatment for their heart problems can be discussed with them.

MEDICAL TREATMENTS FOR HEART DISEASE

A vast array of treatments is now available to deal with heart disease. However, the aim of all of these is to try to restore as effective a blood supply to the heart as possible, and one of the quickest ways of doing this is to keep the blood thin. It may be surprising to learn that one of the best methods is to use one of the oldest drugs we have – aspirin. This not only thins the blood relatively quickly but can be crucial during a heart attack. An aspirin tablet placed under the tongue of someone having an attack often makes the difference between life and death. Aspirin is frequently given along with GTN, which relaxes the body's arteries and veins so that blood supply to the heart is increased. This in turn reduces pressure on the heart and so is very effective in the treatment of angina.

Preventive treatments include beta-blockers, which work by slowing the rate of the heart and improving the efficiency of its pumping, but these can have side effects such as cold extremities and impotence and so must be used with care. Calcium channel blockers also work to reduce the workload of the heart by relaxing blood vessels and both these and beta-blockers may be used to treat high blood pressure as well as angina. To reduce cholesterol levels, a group of drugs known as statins are the current favoured option and are often dramatically effective even at low doses. Most of my patients leaving hospital after either significant angina or a heart attack will have been put on a combination of aspirin, beta-blocker and a statin during their stay and there is now talk of combining these in a 'super pill', although this may not happen for a number of years.

HEART SURGERY

In the main surgical intervention is necessary when medication alone is not effective at relieving symptoms. Among the procedures used are angioplasty, insertion of a pacemaker and, much less commonly, heart transplant.

In angioplasty, in the same way that an angiogram is performed, a small catheter is inserted into the arm or groin under local anaesthetic and threaded up towards the coronary arteries. Once this has reached the point of blockage, a small balloon is inflated which not only pushes open the plaque but also widens the artery and so helps restore normal circulation to the heart. Angioplasty is often effective in the short or medium term, but if the blockage is too severe for this operation to be of use, coronary artery bypass grafting is required. This involves taking veins from the thigh and leg and grafting them around the affected area of the heart. The procedure is now viewed as routine and in experienced hands carries an extremely low mortality rate.

Just as effective is insertion of a pacemaker, which is used if the heart is so diseased that the heartbeat is very erratic or weak. This device, among the most technologically advanced tools we currently have in medicine, sends out permanent currents to stimulate the heart. Pacemakers can now be programmed to automatically speed up the heart rate during exercise and are being increasingly used as the technology continues to improve.

A heart transplant, in which the entire heart is replaced, is reserved for patients for whom all other options have failed and whose quality of life is so poor, or who are so at risk, that transplant is the only option to extend their life long term.

Later in this book I'll look at what I believe to be the best diet in the world to help with heart disease, as well as how to stop smoking, what exercise to take to keep weight down and which natural treatments may help reduce your risk of developing problems with your heart.

KEY POINTS

- Each year five people in every 1,000 in the UK suffer a heart attack and most of these are men.
- Heart attack remains one of the commonest causes of death in the world.
- The majority of heart attacks could have been prevented.

RISK FACTORS
- A family history of heart disease or other precipitating conditions
- High blood pressure
- High cholesterol levels
- Diabetes
- Excessive weight
- A high-fat diet
- Smoking
- Excessive consumption of alcohol
- Lack of exercise

DANGER SIGNS
- Central chest pain, sometimes spreading to the arms, neck or jaw
- Breathlessness
- Anxiety, restlessness, nausea and belching
- Chest pain on exertion or in cold weather
- Severe tiredness after exertion
- Palpitations

2
BLOOD PRESSURE

'Stiffen the sinews, summon up the blood.'
– **Henry V**, *Act 3*

If I had a pound for every time I've checked someone's blood pressure, I'd now be sitting on a beach in Barbados, leading a life of luxury. Unfortunately, such monetary munificence has passed me by and so I continue in my role as a happy, plodding family doctor.

Meanwhile it remains a fact that in the UK about half of all men between 55 and 65 have high blood pressure, or what is more correctly called hypertension. There are a great many myths and old wives' tales about what blood pressure is and why high blood pressure can be harmful. Topping the list of these is the notion that it is only frantically busy, nervous and high-profile types who suffer from it. On the contrary, very calm and laid-back people are just as likely to be affected, but whether you are stressed out or chilled out, one of the problems with high blood pressure is that it is often 'silent', which means it displays no symptoms. It has been estimated that at least a third of people who have blood pressure higher than is good for them are blissfully unaware of the fact. As a result high blood pressure has been dubbed 'the silent killer' and there is no question that it is one of the most serious health problems facing men over 50.

The reason for this is that sustained hypertension not only puts strain on the heart and circulation, but also leads to problems with the kidneys, eyes and limbs. Although high blood pressure is readily treatable, the trick here is to diagnose and treat it before serious complications have arisen, since once these occur they are usually there to stay.

WHAT IS BLOOD PRESSURE?

The heart is essentially a pump. Like any pump, it has to exert pressure to move fluid around a circulation system – in our case blood around the body. Every cell of the body needs a steady supply of blood in order to receive the oxygen and nutrients it requires, and blood can only reach all of our cells if it is driven by a steady pressure. As with simple plumbing, the pressure within our blood vessels depends on the force and quantity of blood coming from the pump. Rather like a tap that is repeatedly turned on and off, the heart constantly pumps through regular cycles of contraction and relaxation. As a result the blood in our bodies is under different pressures depending on whether the heart is in the contracting or the relaxing phase. Contraction is known as systole and relaxation as diastole. Systolic pressure and diastolic pressure are measured in millimetres of mercury, and the first is always higher. Doctors describe blood pressure, for example, as a systolic pressure of 120mm Hg and a diastolic pressure of 80mm Hg, which is written as 120/80. The ideal blood pressure does not exist, but a healthy range in adults extends from 120/70 to 140/85.

There are two main systems in the body which are responsible for day-to-day maintenance of blood pressure. The first is the heart and circulation, known together as the cardiovascular system. The amount of blood that the heart pumps, the force with which it pumps and the size of the blood vessels it pumps blood through all have an effect on blood pressure. This system can react to changing circumstances, for example exercise, by increasing the speed and power of the heart, expanding and contracting the walls of arteries and veins and reducing blood flow to organs that are not critical during exercise, such as the stomach and liver.

The other system which regulates blood pressure is the kidneys. These play a vital role in its control because their basic function is to filter waste products and excess salt and water out of our bodies in the form of urine. If these remain in our blood, they increase the blood volume and so elevate blood pressure. So if there is a problem with the kidneys which hinders waste removal, blood pressure can rise.

Readings of systolic and diastolic pressure, conventionally grouped as below, are in my view slightly artificial, but they can be useful in helping to determine the degree of treatment required.

Systolic	Diastolic	Condition
130-139	85-89	Normal blood pressure
140-159	90-99	Mild hypertension
160-179	100-109	Moderate hypertension
180-209	110-119	Severe hypertension
210 or higher	120 or higher	Very severe hypertension

Although there are certain risk factors which predispose a person to high blood pressure, such as obesity and smoking, in 90% of patients with the condition there is no known cause. It simply happens. This type of blood pressure is known as primary or essential hypertension. In the relatively small number of people whose blood pressure is raised as the result of another illness or condition, high blood pressure is known as secondary hypertension. Among the causes are kidney disorders, diabetes, hormonal problems and pregnancy.

Most experts now believe that the main cause of essential hypertension is a gradual narrowing of the arteries as the result of a build-up of fatty deposits in the blood vessel walls. Imagine slowly narrowing a garden hose as water goes through it. The pressure of fluid going through the hose increases, and this is an exact analogy of what happens in our bodies. This high pressure affects all our tissues, but our kidneys and eyes are most at risk as the fine blood vessels they contain are prone to leak under strain and this damages these organs.

General risk factors that may predispose you to having high blood pressure include:

- A family history of high blood pressure.
- Being a man. Up to the age of 55 more men than women in the UK have high blood pressure but after this age women rapidly catch up.
- Getting older. As we age our blood vessels become less elastic, although the harmful effects this may cause can be mitigated by exercise and healthy eating.
- Diet. Too much salt or potassium in our food can raise blood pressure, as can too little calcium. Rather more recently alcohol has been thrown into the mix, and although the evidence is conflicting (moderate drinkers of alcohol are probably least at risk here), if you already have high blood pressure, drinking too much can raise it a good deal more.

- Smoking. No matter how little you smoke, bear in mind that every cigarette causes blood vessels to constrict, which, in turn, can exacerbate high blood pressure.
- A sedentary lifestyle. A lack of physical activity has a knock-on effect on problems such as obesity, high cholesterol levels and lack of heart fitness. These are all predisposing factors.
- Stress. A contentious issue. Acute stress, such as may occur before a job interview or an exam, does raise the blood pressure but is usually transient, and levels return to normal soon afterwards. This does not cause problems but longer-term stress may consistently cause blood pressure to elevate, although much more research is needed in this area. Studies have shown that people in top management positions have lower blood pressure than those on the shop floor. It seems that this may be linked to stress caused by lack of control in the workplace and poor pay, as well as by smoking and diet.

SIGNS AND SYMPTOMS OF HIGH BLOOD PRESSURE

A silent killer is exactly that – silent. It is tragic that many people do not realise that they are suffering from high blood pressure until they suffer a serious heart attack or a stroke. Some figures have suggested that less than a third of people with hypertension are actually being treated. Although one can argue with this estimate, it is certainly true that an enormous number of people in this country have high blood pressure but do not realise it.

In some cases symptoms do occur, and there are a number of common ones that can lead to the diagnosis, including:

- Tiredness
- Blurred vision
- Confusion
- Anxiety
- Nausea and vomiting
- Sweating
- Flushing of the face
- Chest pain
- Nosebleed
- Palpitations
- Noises in the ears
- Throbbing in the head or headaches

In the absence of signs of high blood pressure, the only way of knowing whether yours is normal or not is to have it measured.

There are natural ways of reducing high blood pressure. For many people simple lifestyle changes alone can be enough to bring their blood pressure down to normal levels, so medication is by no means needed in every case. But lifestyle must be viewed as a whole, rather than simply focusing on one aspect. In this way not only will blood pressure have a chance of returning to normal but long-term health will greatly improve as well. Regular exercise is important, as is watching what you eat and, if necessary, losing weight. It can also be helpful to reduce your daily levels of stress by using complementary therapies such as yoga, acupuncture or meditation, which are discussed in greater detail in the chapter on stress. Keeping to the approved levels of alcohol is sensible, and here a good guide for a man is no more than two drinks a day. Although smoking itself does not cause high blood pressure, it undoubtedly makes it worse and increases the risks the condition poses, so it should be stopped, however many or few cigarettes are smoked.

TESTING FOR HIGH BLOOD PRESSURE

Everyone over 50 should have their blood pressure checked at least once a year. This is done very simply and although this task has always been carried out by GPs, all healthcare professionals are now trained to do it. A huge range of home testing kits and portable machines is also available. The apparatus used to test blood pressure is a sphygmomanometer, which is a cuff that is fitted around the upper arm and inflated to a pressure high enough to temporarily stop the blood flow through the arm. The pressure in the cuff is then slowly lowered until the blood begins to flow again and the arm pulse can be detected with either a stethoscope or an automated blood pressure monitor. This reading is the systolic pressure.

The pressure in the sphygmomanometer is then lowered further until the pulse can no longer be heard, and this is the diastolic pressure. It is very important to realise that blood pressure varies naturally over a 24-hour period, being generally highest when we get up and lowest at three or four in the morning. As a result one-off readings can be notoriously inaccurate, so I never personally take these as gospel. I prefer to either have a series of readings done at different times or for the patient to wear a 24-hour blood pressure ambulatory monitor, which allows fluctuations in blood pressure to be monitored during work, sleep and exercise. This is especially good if someone is very anxious or experiences 'white-coat hypertension', where the blood pressure test itself causes sufficient anxiety to raise it. If high blood pressure is confirmed, this is often followed up with some other simple investigations, such as a chest X-ray, an ECG to assess the regularity of the heartbeat and whether the heart is under strain, analysis of the urine to look for diabetes or kidney problems and blood tests to also check kidney function as well as cholesterol levels.

If the hypertension is thought to be secondary, other tests can be performed, including X-rays of the kidneys, ultrasound scans of the kidneys and surrounding areas and blood tests for hormonal imbalances.

When I was a medical student it was thought that the diastolic pressure was the most critical figure in determining whether hypertension was present. It is now realised that, even when the diastolic pressure is normal, a consistently high systolic pressure is dangerous, especially in older people.

TREATMENTS FOR HIGH BLOOD PRESSURE

If lifestyle changes fail to have the desired effect, medication will be needed to help control high blood pressure. Five main classes of drugs are currently used to treat hypertension, often in combination. The preferred method of treatment is to give two or three low-dose drugs rather than one drug in large doses. The classes of medicines used are:

- Diuretics such as Bendrofluazide. These act to remove salt and water from the circulation and so lower the blood volume.
- Beta-blockers such as Propanolol. These slow down the tendency of the blood vessels to constrict, as well as slowing the heart rate and reducing the force of the heart's contraction.

- ACE (angiotensin converting enzyme) inhibitors such as Ramipril. These act on the kidneys and inhibit the enzyme cascade, which is responsible for the body's retention of water and salt. As a result blood pressure is lowered.
- Calcium channel blockers such as Amlodipine. These work by reducing the force of the heart's contraction and the constriction of blood vessels in general.
- Alpha-blockers such as Prazosin. These work by dilating arteries and veins throughout the body.

All of these drugs have side effects and must be used with caution in certain groups of patients. Indeed everyone needs treatment tailored to them alone, so discuss with your doctor which type is likely to be best for you.

LOW BLOOD PRESSURE

I'm surprised at how often I'm asked if there is any treatment for low blood pressure, or hypotension, and whether the condition is a problem. The medical advice is that in general the lower the blood pressure the better, and in most people it rarely falls below 90/60. Hypotension is usually the result of a reduction in blood volume caused by sweating after exercise or in hot weather, shock, pregnancy, or drinking or eating irregularly. For most people, suffering from low blood pressure is a transient problem and symptoms include feeling faint on standing or getting out of bed. This is known as postural hypotension and is harmless unless fainting occurs often and becomes a problem. To reduce the risk of postural hypotension, sit on the side of the bed before getting out, and when standing up from a sitting position put your hand on a solid object to steady yourself.

If you have low blood pressure the simplest way of raising it is to drink plenty of fluids through the day to increase your blood volume, and especially during or after exercise.

KEY POINTS

- High blood pressure is one of the biggest risk factors in the health of men over 50.
- It is usually 'silent' or has few symptoms.
- Most cases have no proven cause.
- Most cases can be improved with simple lifestyle changes.
- When treatment is needed it is usually for life.
- The only way of knowing your blood pressure is to have it measured. How you feel is irrelevant as most people with hypertension feel well.
- Low blood pressure is not a serious problem, but if it causes loss of balance or fainting it can easily be raised to remedy these.

3
DIABETES

'Sound health is like true friendship; the value of it is seldom known until it is lost.'
– Anonymous

Over the past decade what I've noticed, perhaps more than any other change, it is that the number of diabetic patients on my list has grown inexorably. If I were an economist I would say they are far outstripping the rate of inflation. In other words I'm seeing, year on year, more and more patients with recently diagnosed diabetes than I would expect. Top of the pack here seem to be men and especially men over 50, which is why this is such a crucial chapter in this book. A great deal of myth and misunderstanding surrounds diabetes, not least the fact that there are two distinct types of diabetes, which are often treated slightly differently. Nevertheless, in most of my men (and women) over 50 there is one factor that crops up time and time again and at which I have to point the finger as a major cause in the development of diabetes – weight.

Although there are a number of reasons for obesity, the fact remains that we are turning into a nation of fatties. Excessive weight can have such a dramatic effect on the development of diabetes that simple weight loss is often one of the recommended first treatments for diabetes in older people. In fact, I would go as far as to say that many cases of diabetes in the over-50s would have been preventable by weight loss alone.

WHAT IS DIABETES?

If I were to toddle down my local high street and ask a hundred people what diabetes is, most of them would say something along the lines of 'A bit too much sugar' or 'It's something to do with eating too many sweets and chocolates.' In other words many people know that sugar is involved somewhere but have a rather hazy idea of the role it plays. To put it simply, diabetes is a condition in which the body loses its ability to regulate and control the glucose levels in the blood. As a result diabetics have abnormally high levels of blood glucose, more often called blood sugar, which causes them significant health problems. In someone like me, who does not have diabetes, blood sugar levels are controlled by insulin, a hormone which is vital for life. Insulin is produced by the pancreas, a gland in the middle of the body, and regulates the passage of glucose into our cells, which use it to fuel our bodies. In diabetes, however, one of three things can happen:

- The insulin that is produced does not work as well as it should. This is rather like running your car on two-star petrol instead of four-star.
- Insufficient insulin is produced to cope with the blood sugar levels.
- The body completely stops making insulin.

This is where the two different types of diabetes can be distinguished. In Type 1 (or insulin-dependent) diabetes the body stops making any insulin at all, a condition which occurs most often in young people. In Type 2 (or non-insulin dependent) diabetes insulin is produced but the amount is insufficient or the quality poor. The disease tends to affect the middle-aged, the elderly and the overweight.

When we have abnormally high levels of sugar in our blood, the body's natural reaction is to try to pass it out in the urine, which is why one of the symptoms of diabetes is a need to urinate far more frequently than normal.

Both types of diabetes are such an important health issue because, if left untreated, they can lead to serious health problems, including blindness, accelerated heart disease, kidney failure, stroke, nerve damage and ultimately death. The good news, though, is that these complications can be avoided by early diagnosis, alteration in lifestyle and effective treatment.

WHO IS AT RISK?

Although the exact cause of diabetes remains somewhat shrouded in mystery, like so many medical conditions it is probably the result of a combination of environmental and genetic factors. The scale of the problem can be seen by the fact that at least three in every hundred people in the UK will develop diabetes and there are nearly 1.5 million people who have been diagnosed with the disease. This is significant enough, but even more worrying is the fact that it has been estimated that almost the same number of people are diabetic but are blissfully unaware of it. It is this enormous pool of undiagnosed people who are most at risk and whom doctors are desperately trying to get hold of to treat.

There are, though, clear risk factors for diabetes and the common ones I see include:

- Being a man. Men are at least one and a half times more likely to develop diabetes than women. My view is that this is partially linked to the following factor.
- Weight and shape. At least 80% of my Type 2 diabetic patients are fat. The more overweight someone and the more sedentary their lifestyle, the greater the risk of developing diabetes. There is one body shape that appears more predisposed than all others to developing Type 2 diabetes. This is obesity of the 'big belly' or 'beer belly' kind, where the bulk of the body's fat is deposited around the waist.
- Family history. The more close relatives you have with diabetes the greater the risk you have of developing it yourself. Although only 10% of Type 1 diabetics have a significant family history of diabetes, at least one-third of Type 2 diabetics have a close relative with the condition.
- Age. The older you are the greater the risk. A fact which won't escape this book's target readership is that the average age of diagnosis for Type 2 diabetes is 52 years in those with no family history or 50 in those with a family history. After 75 the risk factor appears to flatten out slightly, so I tend to think that 50–75 is the most dangerous time for Type 2 diabetes.
- Ethnic background. People of Asian or Afro-Caribbean origin living in the UK are some five times more likely to develop diabetes than their Caucasian equivalents. In fact, although Type 2 diabetes generally affects people over 40, it often occurs in Asian and Afro-Caribbean people younger than this.

WHAT'S THE DIFFERENCE?

Although it is Type 2 diabetes that is most often found in men over 50, it is worth looking in more detail at the difference between the two types as this helps us to understand some of the problems that need to be dealt with. As we have seen, Type 1 diabetics lose the ability to make any insulin themselves in their bodies. Although this form of the disease can occur at any age, it is much more common in children and people under the age of 40. In young people the condition becomes evident very quickly and can, in fact, be a medical emergency.

In Type 2 diabetes, which is the form seen in at least 75% of diabetics of both sexes, age is a more relevant factor and so this is often known as late-onset or mature-onset diabetes. It develops much more slowly than Type 1, so symptoms are less obvious, which is why so many people are walking about with the condition without knowing it. As their diabetes gradually develops over a period of months or years they put the way they are feeling down to factors such as age, weight, lack of fitness, or just think, this is simply how I'm feeling and that's that. It is a salutary thought that it has been estimated that on average people will have Type 2 diabetes for six or seven years before they are diagnosed. I often see people who refer to Type 2 diabetes as being mild or having 'a touch of diabetes', and this is worrying. There is no mild form of diabetes – all types must be viewed as potentially dangerous. Just because you don't need insulin injections to control your blood sugar levels, it does not mean that complications and risks don't exist.

WHAT ARE THE SYMPTOMS?

Fortunately, there are many common symptoms in someone with untreated diabetes. So if you know what you are looking for, you can easily investigate the possibility that you are diabetic and then, if appropriate, get a full medical test. In no particular order, the symptoms I see time and again are:

- Tiredness, fatigue and lethargy.
- Increased thirst, sometimes so intense that it can't be quenched no matter how much fluid is drunk.
- The need to urinate constantly, including getting out of bed repeatedly at night to do so.
- Recurrent infections of the skin, such as boils or spots.
- Blurred vision or problems with focusing, both of which may vary during the day.
- General itchiness, but especially around the genitals.
- Weight loss. This is particularly common in Type 1 diabetes, although it occurs in both types and can happen even when there is an increased appetite.

Fortunately, the diagnosis of diabetes is easily made. This can be done by either a simple dip test of the urine to show the presence of sugar in the blood, or a finger-prick blood test or a fasting blood sugar level test to show high levels of blood sugar.

TREATMENT OF DIABETES

The treatment of diabetes is a rapidly expanding area, with new developments coming on to the scene all the time. There are two treatments that I recommend above all others for my diabetic patients. The first is a combination of sensible eating and regular exercise. The second is medication, in the form of tablets or insulin or both. Whatever the treatment, every diabetic patient needs to be assessed individually and treatment is for life. This second point is particularly important, because some people believe that once you have brought sugar levels down to where they should be you can waltz off and carry on as if nothing had happened. I wish that were the case, but it isn't. Once it exists diabetes can't be cured, but it can be treated for the rest of the patient's life.

Nevertheless, diabetes is a progressive condition, which means that its natural tendency is to worsen over time. Therefore the aim of treatment is to slow any such progression. Recent research has shown repeatedly that the sooner medication and treatment are started, the less likely the patient is to develop complications in later life. Let's now look at what kind of treatment is given for the disease.

● **Type 1 diabetes.** The treatment here is insulin. Type 1 diabetics must have insulin every day of their lives and this requirement is non-negotiable. Unfortunately, insulin is very quickly destroyed by the acid and digestive juices found in our stomachs, which is why it can't be taken as a tablet but has to be injected. Typically, insulin is injected between two and four times a day, although the recent development of the once-daily, long-acting insulin Glargine has revolutionised the treatment of many Type 1 diabetics. Although insulin injections are very effective, this does not mean that Type 1 diabetics should not continue to eat a healthy diet and keep physically active – indeed these measures are still crucial. New research shows that it is vitally important to keep not

41

only blood sugar levels well controlled but also blood pressure levels, and for this reason many diabetic patients, of Type 1 and Type 2, need treatment to control their blood pressure as strictly as possible.

Needle phobia is nowadays acknowledged far more readily by doctors than it was in the past, but it still remains a problem for some patients. However, it is no longer a reason for not complying with insulin treatment. With the advent of high-tech, compressed air-based injections, no needle is used, and previously anxious patients report far greater control of their diabetes when using these. Although this option is not yet widely available on the NHS, in time more and more insulin-dependent diabetics will be able to access it if appropriate.

● **Type 2 diabetes.** There are a number of ways in which Type 2 diabetes can be managed and to some extent the treatment depends on how severe it had become before diagnosis. A healthy diet, low in sugar and rich in fresh fruit and vegetables, when combined with regular exercise and weight loss, can be enough to keep blood glucose levels acceptable. However, for the majority of Type 2 diabetics such a healthy diet and physical activity must be allied to either tablets or tablets and insulin injections. The tablets (known as oral hypoglycaemic agents or OHAs) work in one of three ways. They help more insulin to be produced by the body, improve the body's use of the insulin that is produced or slow down the speed at which the body absorbs sugar from the gut.

People with either type of diabetes are also more likely to have increased blood pressure and cholesterol levels, in which case these problems will need attention as well, either in the form of diet or tablets. I've occasionally heard a newly diagnosed diabetic patient say somewhat ruefully that they walked into my office feeling generally unwell but not desperately ill, only to walk out diagnosed with diabetes and other conditions, and enough pills to make them rattle. It is crucial that the whole of a diabetic patient is treated and not necessarily just the blood sugar.

General practitioners now almost universally run diabetic clinics in their practices and there is an increasing emphasis on diabetic patients being seen routinely in clinic rather than in hospital. The purpose of routine check-ups is to make sure that treatment is progressing satisfactorily and that complications are not developing. The goal of treatment is always to continue a normal daily life while controlling the blood sugar satisfactorily. To take an extreme example to make my point, perhaps one of the most inspirational figures for diabetics of all ages is Sir Steve Redgrave, who, even though he is a Type 1 diabetic, is possibly our greatest-ever Olympian, with five Olympic gold medals to his credit. There are dozens of other examples of well-known sportsmen and high achievers who are at the top of their particular tree despite their diabetes.

HELPING YOURSELF

Whether you are newly diagnosed or have been diabetic for many years, there are five important habits you need to get into, then stick to, in order to help yourself cope with this long-term condition:

● **Follow a healthy diet.** I tend not to advise a set 'diabetic diet' as all diabetic patients are different and respond in individual ways to what they eat, but basic dietary principles apply here. Cutting out all the obvious sugar from the diet is the first thing to do, and I'm sorry to say this means cakes, biscuits, pastries and sweets. Alcohol should be kept to a minimum, fresh food is the order of the day, to reduce the amount of processed sugar and salt-rich foods being eaten, and eating plenty of fruit and vegetables every day is also important. We also need to remember that our body metabolism progressively slows by 3% each decade and so the calorific content of food needs to be checked more carefully anyway. Many men find that between 50 and 65 their sense of taste alters, with the result that they believe they need more salt or sugar in food, but a healthier option here is to use spices or herbs instead. Simple measures can have radically beneficial results, so eat as naturally as possible, eat small meals regularly to keep blood sugar levels as stable as possible, and avoid caffeine, which, like refined sugar and alcohol, robs the body of vital nutrients such as B vitamins.

Use the following as a checklist for your diet:

- Reduce your intake of processed foods.
- Avoid yo-yo dieting at all costs as this will only increase weight over the years.
- Drink at least eight glasses of water every day.
- Eat five portions of fresh fruit and vegetables every day.
- Eat bread, rice, fortified cereal or pasta every day.
- Eat fats, oils and sweets sparingly.
- Take calcium supplements and multivitamins to ensure there is no dietary deficiency.

Some diabetics find it a battle to lose weight and this is sometimes because they have other health problems that make it difficult to exercise. I've lost count of the number of patients who have looked at me aghast when I weigh them and point out that they have put weight on rather than taken it off. Their protests of innocence would carry more clout with me if I had not seen them down the pub or in the chip shop that same week! We all have considerable ability to delude ourselves as to how much food actually goes into our mouths each day. Keeping an honest food diary can be very illuminating and I would recommend doing this for a week or two. The key word here is 'honest' – if you cheat, the only person who will suffer is you. Make a record of absolutely everything you eat and drink, and when. See if patterns of eating develop, if you comfort-eat or if you tend to eat the same unhealthy foods at particular times. You may be surprised.

● **Quit smoking.** If I've heard one diabetic patient say to me that smoking is their last pleasure, so why should they give it up, I've heard it a hundred times. Unfortunately, smoking and diabetes go together like petrol and matches since the habit dramatically accelerates the development of heart disease in diabetics. If you are diabetic and smoke, turn to the chapter on smoking and see how you can quit *now*.

● **Get physical.** You do not have to be like Steve Redgrave and row a boat at Olympic level to get fit, but the fitter you are the easier it is to control your diabetes. This can be done as simply as by walking for 30 minutes a day, and a very big American study recently confirmed the fact. The study looked at people who took a brisk half-hour walk every day and it found that, regardless of age or body weight, men and women who were physically active like this for at least 30 minutes each day were less likely to develop diabetes. No great surprise there, but, by contrast with previous studies that have investigated the link between physical activity and diabetes risk, at the end of the process participants were tested for the presence of diabetes by a formal glucose test rather than by self-reporting. Just under 2,000 men and women aged between 15 and 60 were followed for six years, with a high proportion of these being American Indians, who traditionally have a high rate of diabetes. During the study nearly 350 of these people developed Type 2 diabetes, but the more physically active the participant, the less likely they were to develop diabetes. Such research has now led the US Surgeon General to recommend that adults engage in at least 30 minutes of moderate physical activity on all or most days of the week.

● **Stick to your treatment plan.** Whether you are on diet alone, tablets, exercise or insulin, never be tempted to miss out on your treatment, even if you are feeling well. The tighter your control is all the time, the greater the benefits in the long term. As I often say to patients, you are putting money in the bank for the long term. Don't be tempted to make a quick withdrawal now that will cause you to suffer later.

● **Have a regular medical check-up.** Everyone with diabetes should have a thorough check-up at least every year so that complications such as eye disease or foot problems can be caught at an early stage before symptoms are apparent and so that treatment can be commenced. The items that should be included in an annual check-up are:

- Blood sugar levels. Included here are checks on cholesterol levels, kidney function and liver function, an ordinary blood count and a check to test the amount of long-term glucose that there has been in the blood. This last test is known as an HbA1c and is a very effective measurement of how well the diabetes is being controlled.
- Blood pressure.
- The presence of protein in the urine (a condition known as albuminuria).
- A foot examination to make sure there is no nerve damage and that the circulation is satisfactory.
- Weight measurement.
- A check on smoking.
- A discussion of lifestyle and exercise habits.

KEY POINTS

- Diabetes affects 2% of the UK population, with possibly as many further cases undiagnosed.
- Diabetes is a major cause of serious illnesses, particularly heart disease, impotence, kidney problems, blindness and stroke.
- Excessive weight is a major risk factor in diabetes.
- The incidence of Type 2 diabetes increases with age.
- The earlier either type of diabetes is diagnosed and correctly treated, the less the risk of serious complications in the future.
- Treatments include tablets, insulin, weight loss, alteration in diet and regular exercise.

DANGER SIGNS

- **Thirst and a constant need to urinate**
- **Tiredness**
- **Weight loss**
- **Spots, skin rashes or boils**
- **Blurred vision**

4
DEPRESSION

'A new study has shown that licking a toad cures depression. The trouble is, once you stop licking, the toad gets depressed again.'
– Jay Leno

If you were one of the first men on the moon, or steered your country to victory in the Second World War, you would expect to be pretty chirpy about life, wouldn't you? Well, despite their amazing and heroic exploits, both Buzz Aldrin and Sir Winston Churchill suffered from depression, with Churchill famously referring to it as his 'black dog' that followed him around constantly. These are not the only famous sufferers – Mozart was almost certainly one, as was Spike Milligan – and a scientific study of almost 300 world-famous men found that over 40% had experienced some type of depression. Famous writers are particularly prone to the problem, but others also suffer high rates of depression – artists, composers, politicians and scientists, for example. I make this point simply to show how anyone can be affected by this most common of mental illnesses, irrespective of intellect, profession, achievement or wealth.

About a quarter of all drugs prescribed by the NHS are for mental health problems and between 1990 and 1995 the number of prescriptions issued by doctors for antidepressants in England rose by over 100%. Although the general public is far more at risk from young men under the influence of alcohol than from any patient with a mental health problem, there is still a great deal of discrimination towards people with mental ill health. The ignorance and insensitivity of this attitude is something I constantly try to inform people of when talking about depression and mental health problems in general.

There is much confusion when people talk about depression and they often use the word incorrectly to describe feeling low or having got out of bed on the wrong side. Depression is not simply feeling unhappy or worried, and it is certainly more serious than feeling blue or down in the dumps for a few days. It is common in people over 50 and in men the highest incidence of first attacks of the illness occurs between the ages of 55 and 65. At any given time one in four people in Britain suffers from some form of depression – a staggering figure – and one in six people who have suffered from depression commit suicide.

The World Health Organisation has estimated that by 2020 depression will be the second most debilitating condition in the developed world, so it is clear just how important it is not only to recognise how and why it occurs but also what can be done about it. Rather shamefully, from my point of view as a doctor, studies show that some 50% of people with clinical depression fail to receive a proper diagnosis or treatment. To me this is simply not acceptable as the vast majority of these can be helped with simple and appropriate advice and treatment.

RISK FACTORS

Depression is a complex disorder in which many different factors may be implicated. The main ones are:

● **Genetics.** There is no question that our genes and family history play an important role in the development of depression. If you have a first-degree relative (such as a parent or brother or sister) with depression, then your risk of developing the condition is between two and three times that of the general population. In addition, the younger the age of onset in that relative, the stronger the genetic influence tends to be. Even so, it is rare for genetic factors alone to trigger clinical depression and many other factors are usually involved.

● **Childhood.** If we leave out of the equation the complex issue of childhood sexual abuse, it may still come as a surprise to many people that there are few proven links between a disadvantaged childhood and depression as an adult. However, there is no question in my mind that a difficult upbringing, poor parenting and lack of emotional support can all be linked to negative thinking in adults, which is a very common feature of depression.

● **Stress.** Time and time again I see stressful events in somebody's life triggering the start of a depressive process. When you quiz depressed people about the number of stressful events in their lives they tend to report more of these than the average person. I'm talking here about stress caused not only by events or situations but also by physical illness, as 5–10% of people with clinical depression link it to a physical problem. In fact, about a quarter of people with heart disease, cancer or diabetes develop depression at some point in their illness.

● **Diet.** In itself diet is not a major trigger for depression. However, we all now eat much more processed food than we used to and many of us rush meals, put up with poor nutrition for convenience and consume a lot of caffeine, all of which can adversely affect our well-being. This, in turn, reduces our ability to deal with stress and negative thoughts. So, although it is not a crucial factor, inadequate diet can be another part of the jigsaw that tips someone over into clinical depression.

● **Social factors.** It seems to be part of a man's make-up to try to be powerful and successful, so when unemployment strikes or a man has a female boss he can feel that his status as a male has been eroded. A man's feeling that his competitive drive is thwarted, and a sense of vulnerability or even uselessness, have been cited as being among the reasons why male depression is on the rise. Another factor may be the fact that nowadays most divorces are initiated by women, and it is well known that divorced men are much more likely than the average person to kill themselves. In all of these situations it is quite common for a man to turn to the bottle to drown his sorrows rather than getting them out in the open, and excessive drinking will itself exacerbate depression. Here we come back to the old chestnut that many men feel that to admit vulnerability is to be weak.

Depression is such a severe illness because, to put it bluntly, it kills people. Nearly three-quarters of the 4,000 suicides in the UK each year are among depressives and three times as many men as women commit suicide. (Many more women than men attempt suicide, but men more often complete the act.) This higher suicide rate among men is reflected all over the world, but even so the reasons why men are more likely to kill themselves remain rather ill defined. However, it is widely agreed that among the key factors are age, with peaks of suicide in the twenties and then between 55 and 70, unemployment – in many countries the suicide rate has been shown to rise and fall with the unemployment rate – and social isolation, as those who kill themselves often live alone.

Chronic physical illness also increases the risk of suicide in men. And then there are certain occupations which ought to carry a health warning here. As a rural GP I'm all too aware that farmers, who usually work alone and have access to shotguns, are at higher risk of suicide. The more severe a depression is the more likely it is to lead to suicide. Here men are certainly more likely to choose decisive methods such as shooting or hanging rather than tablets or cutting their wrists.

It is a sad fact that when depressed men visit their doctor they are more likely to complain of physical symptoms or vague ill health than to say they are feeling depressed or distressed. Moreover, health professionals may, I feel, be less likely to consider a diagnosis of mental illness in a man, while men themselves are less likely than women to recognise when they are under severe stress or depression. This is perhaps illustrated by the fact that about 80% of women who commit suicide consult their doctor in the weeks before their death but only 50% of male suicides do so.

It is important to bear in mind that suicide prompted by depression is avoidable, because the illness is treatable.

WHEN SHOULD YOU SEE A DOCTOR?

An episode of clinical depression can come on over weeks or months, giving the sufferer time to think about seeking help, but it often strikes out of the blue. There are a number of well-recognised symptoms that suggest depression. If you have five or more of the following, especially if they have lasted for more than a fortnight, you should seek medical advice:

- A loss of pleasure or enjoyment of life
- Persistent feelings of unhappiness which refuse to lift and can be worse at certain times of the day, particularly in the early morning
- Blaming yourself for things which you know really have nothing to do with you. These guilt feelings can be very strong.
- A feeling of being useless or worthless
- Memory problems and difficulty in concentrating even on simple tasks
- A loss of appetite or lack of interest in food
- Significant weight loss that can't be explained by diet
- Insomnia. There may be trouble in getting off to sleep or you may wake during the night and be unable to get back to sleep
- Temporary or permanent thoughts of suicide or harming yourself

In addition to these common symptoms you may lose interest in sex, feel irritable and angry for no reason and find it almost impossible to make decisions at work or at home.

A further problem here is that if you are in the grip of a depressive illness, and so have little energy or sense of purpose, you may find it almost impossible to motivate yourself to seek help or even to believe that you are justified in asking for it.

Recent research has suggested that even highly competent doctors can initially miss the diagnosis of depression in about half the cases put in front of them, although this figure falls at the next and subsequent consultations. This may be partly due to the doctor not being tuned in to the often subtle signs and symptoms of the illness, but depressed people can be unintentionally vague about their symptoms, which can make diagnosis much harder.

An area of particular concern is that in later life sufferers can believe that how they are feeling is simply a consequence of getting old, when in fact it is depression that is the main problem. If they are diagnosed accordingly and given appropriate treatment, they are fortunate, but many cases of clinical depression in older people go unidentified.

DIAGNOSIS AND TREATMENT OF DEPRESSION

If I had one simple test, such as a blood test, which could confirm the diagnosis of depression, my life would be hunky-dory. Unfortunately, no such test exists and there is no brain scan or other wondrous device that will provide a diagnosis. This can only be made from the symptoms. Most psychiatrists tell me they will make a diagnosis of depression if someone has a persistently low mood which influences their everyday activities to a considerable degree, which has been present for a minimum of a fortnight and which is associated with at least four of the other common symptoms of depression. Although a physical examination is important and blood tests may be done to rule out other possibilities, such as anaemia or thyroid problems, in most people with depression any tests that are taken turn out to be normal or negative.

There are a number of ways to treat depression and this fact alone may surprise those people who believe that, for whatever reason, their depression is not treatable. Occasionally people slip quietly towards clinical depression, but if they talk about it or discuss their problems with their partner, relatives or friends, this alone can be enough to pull them back from the brink and keep them functioning normally. More formal 'talking therapy', properly described as psychotherapy, has been shown to be as effective as medication for the treatment of mild depression. The biggest advance here has been the development of cognitive behavioural therapy (CBT), which attempts to change the way you feel by changing the way you think. Most people who are depressed have what are called negative automatic thoughts which constantly flick in and out of the mind. These destructive thoughts intrude into normal thinking patterns and make you feel more and more depressed, which in turn increases the amount of negative thinking you do. Some experts have suggested that, even after an initial triggering event has long gone, it is these negative automatic thoughts which keep people in a depressed state of mind, and this is where CBT often comes up with the goods. Therapists encourage the person to think about more reasonable and positive interpretations of circumstances that may have triggered negative thinking. They also get them to rate their anxieties on a floating scale of 1–10 and help them to reduce their anxiety by using simple relaxation techniques.

An overview of many studies of CBT has concluded that in the short term it is at least as effective in treating depressed patients as drugs, that in the long term it often works better and that combining the two treatments is more effective than using either one alone. My problem as a GP is that CBT therapists are like gold dust. This is an area of the NHS that needs a substantial increase in resources, as it is perhaps one of the most cost-effective things that could be done for any condition. But I'm not holding my breath.

MEDICATION

For decades antidepressants have been the mainstay of treatment for most depressed people and are effective for two-thirds of moderate and severe cases. Whenever I prescribe them I always give my little set speech which points out that they are not addictive, they are not sleeping tablets, they are not tranquillisers and they often take two or three weeks to start working effectively. I emphasise also that they are not so-called 'happy pills' and do not change someone's personality. It may seem strange that it is not exactly clear how antidepressants work on the brain, but this is the truth. In general, though, they act on chemicals in the brain to correct underlying abnormalities which help to trigger depression. It is worth adding that new antidepressants are said to have fewer of the side effects which plagued some of the older ones.

The main categories of antidepressants currently used are:

● **Tricyclics.** The granddaddies of antidepressants, these work by raising levels of serotonin and noradrenaline, which are believed to become depleted in people with depression.

Unfortunately, side effects such as weight gain, dizziness and a dry mouth are common, although new drugs in this category have less of these. Examples include Imipramine and Nortriptyline.

● **Monoamine Oxidase Inhibitors (MAOIs).** Again these are old-fashioned drugs, and this group have always been used rather warily because they have been associated with severe side effects when some kinds of food and drink are taken with them, such as cheese and red wine. The more modern MAOIs have far fewer side effects and do work well, although they are not usually the first-line treatment.

● **Specific Serotonin Reuptake Inhibitors (SSRIs).** These are the most frequently prescribed modern anti-depressants and perhaps the best-known example of this group is Prozac (Fluoxetine); others are Paroxetine, Citalopram and Sertraline. SSRIs act on the brain pathways that involve the chemical serotonin and in low doses they are relatively free of side effects. There is no doubt that, if used with care, these can be dramatically effective in treating depression.

● **Noradrenalin Reuptake Inhibitors.** Just as SSRIs work mainly on one brain chemical, these do the same, but here the chemical is noradrenalin. An example is Reboxetine, which, like other drugs in this group, is said to be particularly useful for treating withdrawn or socially crippled depressed patients who are struggling to maintain a job or relationship.

● **Noradrenaline and Serotonin Specific Uptake Inhibitors.** At the cutting edge of depression treatment, these act on both noradrenaline and serotonin while attempting to keep side effects to a minimum. The current favourite prescribed by doctors is Mirtazapine.

There are many things to remember when taking anti-depressant medication, not least the fact that it needs to be taken regularly. Current World Health Organisation guidelines recommend that patients continue to take antidepressants for six months after having recovered, to prevent any recurrence of their illness when the medication is stopped. Although there may be little improvement for a fortnight or so after starting medication, once a response has occurred this should continue to develop over several weeks. Antidepressants can be used both for single episodes of depression and also to prevent further episodes of illness and I often find that patients who have stopped their treatment as soon as they feel better only relapse afterwards. It is best to stop taking the medication only after agreeing this with your doctor, who will advise you to gradually reduce the dose over three to four weeks rather than cease abruptly.

About one in a hundred patients do not respond to straightforward treatment and so require admission to hospital. One possible hospital treatment, which has caused much excitement in the popular press recently, is ECT or electroconvulsive therapy, but this is reserved only for patients with severe depression in whom all other treatments have failed. This involves administering a brief anaesthetic and, while the patient is asleep, a muscle-relaxing drug is given by an anaesthetist and a small electric current is passed through the brain for a fraction of a second. This is often given twice a week, with about half a dozen to a dozen treatments being required to treat depression, although improvement may occur after the first one or two treatments. Given only by a team of anaesthetist, consultant psychiatrist and senior nursing staff, the treatment remains controversial in some quarters but I've absolutely no doubt that it has saved many people's lives and continues to do so. However, many people do not like the idea of ECT, and this is an understandable reaction.

HOW YOU CAN HELP YOURSELF

It is not just a doctor who can help if you are depressed — there are a number of things you can do that can also help to pull you out of this very common illness:

● **Diet.** Make sure you are eating a diet rich in fruit and vegetables as I've often seen depressed patients with very low levels of B vitamins and folic acid. Normally linked to conditions such as heart disease and Alzheimer's disease, low levels of these have now been linked to depression and it is sometimes necessary for doctors to check levels in depressed patients.

● **Exercise.** Although you may not be able to do things you normally would, such as work, keeping active is important as taking physical exercise helps many depressed people. The exact reasons for this are not clear, but my view is that the increased blood flow to the brain during exercise is beneficial. Many doctors are now able to prescribe exercise on prescription, along with psychotherapy or antidepressants, and I'm sure that this combined approach is the way forward.

● **St John's Wort (hypericum).** This is perhaps the best-known herbal remedy used to improve mood and is the only over-the-counter preparation specifically aimed at depression. I've been using this on mildly depressed people for a number of years and have no doubt at all as to its efficacy. Many men with mild depression prefer to try this first, rather than prescription medication. It appears to work by boosting levels of serotonin in the brain in much the same way as modern antidepressants do. Numerous studies have shown the effectiveness of St John's Wort in treating mild depression and seasonal affective disorder (SAD), and it may also help people suffering from stress. However, it should not be taken at the same time as conventional antidepressants and it has little effectiveness in treating moderate to severe depression.

KEY POINTS

- Depression affects at least 20% of people at some time in their life.
- It is common in men over 50.
- It is not a sign of weakness, nor is it something that can be 'snapped out of'.
- It is a dangerous illness as it kills thousands of people each year in the UK alone.
- Treatment is available in the form of cognitive behavioural therapy (CBT) and other forms of psychotherapy, antidepressant medication and, in extreme cases, electroconvulsive therapy.
- A balanced diet and regular exercise often help recovery.

DANGER SIGNS

- A marked loss of enjoyment of life, often with feelings of guilt or unhappiness

- **Poor concentration**
- **Apathy**
- **Tearfulness or emotional sensitivity**
- **Weight loss and lack of appetite**
- **Low sex drive**

5
PROSTATE PROBLEMS

'Nearly all men die of their medicines, not of their diseases.'
– **Molière**

What do Leonardo da Vinci, Bob Monkhouse, Archbishop Desmond Tutu and Emperor Akihito of Japan have in common? The answer is the prostate gland. Nothing earth-shattering there, as being a man does bring with it the requirement of having a prostate gland, but in his beautiful precise anatomical drawings, Leonardo included wonderful examples of every organ, blood vessel and nerve in the human body except for one: the prostate gland. However hard you look at his drawings, you won't find it in any of them, which is quite remarkable when you consider how methodical his dissections were and how precise his drawings. The other three men mentioned have all been diagnosed with prostate cancer and are simply famous names in a long list of men both well known and ordinary who contract or succumb to this disease every year.

It is a sad but true fact that prostate tumours have now become the most commonly diagnosed cancer among men in the UK, having just overtaken lung cancer. Although the figures suggested this would happen at some point, it was not expected to occur until 2005 at the earliest. Whether this means more of us are getting it, or simply that more are being diagnosed with it, is debatable. However, the facts are blunt – 1 in 13 men in this country will be seriously afflicted by prostate disease during their lifetime and over 10,000 die from it every year. Some experts have calculated that prostate cancer will increase by a staggering 47% by 2018, but in my gloomier moments in my surgery I do wonder whether this might actually be an optimistic figure rather than a pessimistic one. I'm sure the situation is not helped by the fact that only about 1% of men currently receive regular prostate check-ups. One reputable poll recently showed that 90% of British men did not know what their prostate gland was, what it did or what warning symptoms it may show. With this level of ignorance, how on earth can I blame my male patients for presenting late with their prostate cancer and so having less chance of successful treatment?

WHAT IS THE PROSTATE GLAND?

The prostate gland is a sexual gland which lies just below the bladder and in front of the rectum, or back passage. It is normally about the size of a walnut and surrounds the tube known as the urethra through which urine flows from the bladder and out of the penis. The gland gradually grows through childhood and puberty to reach its normal adult size. However, from the age of about 45 it again grows larger and as a result can become a source of medical problems both harmless and serious.

Its role is to manufacture an important part of the seminal fluid, which is mixed with sperm and ejaculated at orgasm. Fluid contained in the prostate increases the liquidity of the sperm, which allows it to move more freely and so increases its chances of fertilising the egg. This fluid also contains prostate specific antigen (PSA), which I will be discussing in detail later in the chapter.

Because of where the prostate gland lies, the bladder and urinary system are the principal area that it affects if it starts to malfunction. There are three main diseases of the prostate: prostatitis, benign prostatic hypertrophy (BPH) and prostate cancer.

PROSTATITIS

Perhaps the least common and least well-known prostate problem, prostatitis is inflammation of the area surrounding the prostate gland. It affects more young and middle aged men than elderly men, is responsible for a substantial amount of absence from work and is a source of misery to a great many patients. The term literally means inflammation of the prostate, but this is something of a misnomer as we now know that not every man who has the condition actually has an inflamed prostate. The cause of prostatitis is often unclear, but there are certain groups who are at high risk of developing it. These include men who have had a catheter in place for a long time and men suffering from untreated urinary infections or chronic cystitis. Although men of any age can be affected, the years between 30 and 50 seem to be the peak period for the disease to occur. Most of the men I see with the problem appear to have no identifiable risk factors, although unprotected anal intercourse is definitely one.

The symptoms of prostatitis are a high temperature with a chill or fever, pain, especially felt between the anus and the scrotum (often causing severe discomfort on sitting) and sometimes in the testicles and lower back as well. Some men have told me that their lower back pain is particularly bad just after they have had sex. There may be pain or discomfort, as well as difficulty, in passing urine, and it may become necessary to do so frequently.

Because prostatitis is often the result of a bacterial infection, a number of tests can be done, including urine tests, blood tests and obtaining samples of prostate secretions. A slightly newer test is the Doppler probe, in which an ultrasound of the prostate performed via the rectum can show increased blood flow to the prostate gland, a possible indication of prostatitis.

If bacterial infection is found, antibiotics are the drug of choice. However, a problem for many men is that the medication often needs to be taken for a very long time and compliance is very important since if it is stopped too early some bacteria will remain, divide and grow and so the next infection will be more difficult to treat. If bacteria do not appear to be present, anti-inflammatory drugs can help, often in conjunction with antibiotics, although why these are sometimes effective in the apparent absence of bacteria remains baffling.

Fortunately, prostatitis is not a life-threatening condition and never turns into prostate cancer or BPH. Because this is the least understood of the three common prostate problems it is hardly surprising that we do not yet know how to prevent it. Having your urine tested at the first sign of infection is sensible, as is maintaining a healthy lifestyle, taking regular exercise and avoiding anything that seems to make the problem worse. We still don't know why young men appear to be slightly more prone to this than the elderly.

I've heard of some doctors advising patients with prostatitis to take zinc and high doses of vitamins D and E, but I've found little hard evidence to support this. Finally, it is clear that there is little reason to treat your sexual partner if you develop it.

BENIGN PROSTATIC HYPERTROPHY (BPH)

If there is one phrase that seems to be accepted more than any other with a shrug of the shoulders and a wry smile by my male patients over the age of 50, it is the term 'old man's prostate'. The correct term is benign prostatic hypertrophy (BPH), a condition that arises as a simple consequence of excessive but not cancerous growth of the prostate gland. You will remember that the urethral passage from the bladder to the penis runs through the prostate gland and so if the prostate becomes enlarged the urethra is squeezed and the flow of urine starts to be obstructed. Prostate enlargement is said to affect some 45% of men over 65. No prizes for guessing that the larger the prostate the greater the risk of BPH occurring, but men whose urine naturally tends to flow slowly may also become more likely to develop complications as they age. The classic symptoms of BPH are:

● A weak stream of urine
● Straining to pass urine and urination taking a long time
● Stop/start urination where the urine flow appears to have finished and then restarts (this is known as hesitancy)
● Frequent urination during both the day and night, and an urgent need to pass urine, sometimes with a little leaking at the first sign of wanting to go
● A gradually increasing inability to pass water normally

When presented with a patient with these symptoms, a doctor should make a general physical examination, including of the abdomen, to see whether the bladder is enlarged, and also a digital rectal examination (DRE). Many men are terrified of a DRE, but although it can be slightly uncomfortable, it is brief and enables the doctor to have an idea of the size and consistency of the prostate gland. It also allows them to feel whether the gland is harmless or malignant. Blood and urine tests are also often standard, and more specialised tests will include a urine flow test to measure the speed of urine output over time and ultrasound scans to measure whether urine is being left in the bladder. Other less common tests that specialists may want to perform include urodynamic measurements, where the pressure is measured in the bladder to determine whether symptoms are due to BPH or bladder problems, and trans-rectal ultrasummography (TRUS), used to assess the proportion of the prostate gland and to allow a biopsy if required.

BPH can readily be treated with either drugs or surgery, and if symptoms are mild a wait-and-see approach may be the most sensible option once it has been confirmed that the prostate problem is harmless. If symptoms are moderate, drug treatment is usually the preferred choice of treatment. Here there are two main tools in my kit. The first is alpha-blockers, a class of drugs which work by helping to relax the muscles around the prostate and in the neck of the bladder. Although these do not actually cure BPH, they can be dramatically effective in alleviating symptoms and studies suggest that at least half of all men find their symptoms have greatly improved in the first fortnight of treatment. As with all drugs, alpha-blockers may have side effects, and these affect 10% of all men taking them. Common problems I see include dizziness, headache and tiredness, but some of the more modern alpha-blockers have fewer side effects than the earlier ones.

The second type of drugs are called 5-alpha reductase inhibitors and these work by blocking the conversion of the male hormone testosterone to dihydrotestosterone, which seems to play a key role in enlargement of the prostate gland. These drugs work well, but the side effects can be more troubling than those of alpha-blockers and include erection problems and reduced libido, although these affect a smaller number of men.

BPH can also be treated surgically, and the three options are: TURP – trans-urethral resection of the prostate; TUIP – trans-urethral incision of the prostate; and open prostatectomy.

The most common of these operations is TURP, which is carried out under a general anaesthetic and involves passing a small cutting instrument up through the penis to remove the middle of the enlarged prostate. At the end of the operation a catheter is placed into the bladder to allow urine to pass and this tends to be left in place for a couple of days. This operation is normally very effective, but there may be a burning sensation when passing water, as well as bleeding for some time, after the catheter has been removed. The commonest side effect of a TURP is retrograde ejaculation, whereby semen passes into the bladder at orgasm rather than being expelled from the penis. This means that the next time you pass water semen is passed out as well as urine, but this is not harmful and most men do not find it a problem once they know what is happening. After a TURP some men notice that their bladder control is not as good as it was before, but in the vast majority of cases this improves with time.

A TUIP is usually more appropriate for a man who has BPH but whose prostate is relatively small. The principle is similar to that of a TURP, but rather than a section of the prostate gland being cut away, one or two small cuts are made in the prostate and the neck of the bladder itself. The aim is to allow the bladder neck to open and reduce any obstruction there. Again catheterisation follows the operation. Retrograde ejaculation is much less of a problem here, but if symptoms return in the future a TURP is the usual next step.

An open prostatectomy is the least common surgical option for BPH and is best reserved for men whose prostate gland is very large or who have large stones in the bladder. It is a bigger and more complex procedure than either a TURP or TUIP, with a greater risk of complications. Here the central part of the prostate is removed through a cut in the abdomen and a catheter is inserted to drain urine for several days. The recovery time following this procedure is normally longer than with the other operations, but in almost all men the symptoms improve dramatically. This operation also makes it less likely that further surgery will be needed later.

Somewhat frustratingly, our understanding of BPH allows us to glimpse the hormones testosterone and oestrogen at work in some way here. Studies suggest that men in the Far East appear to have less chance of developing BPH compared with men in the West, and there has been speculation about whether the diet they eat (for example soya, which contains oestrogen-like chemicals) could be protecting them to some degree. The jury is still out on this possibility, but it promises to be an exciting area of research for the future.

PROSTATE CANCER

We now get to the point where many men would prefer to stick their head in the sand and hope that they can avoid thinking about the issue, even when they have started to develop worrying symptoms. Like other cancers, prostate cancer is a disease of the body's cells and occurs when the natural repair and growth of prostate cells becomes uncontrolled. This causes the formation of a tumour, but because prostate cancer can grow very slowly it may take several years for the symptoms to appear and indeed in some men cancers may grow for up to ten years before this happens. I've seen a number of men with prostate cancer who showed no symptoms at all and who only realised the disease was present when it had spread to surrounding tissue walls and caused other symptoms, such as bone pain, to occur. About 60% of men with this cancer have secondary tumours at the time of diagnosis.

Prostate cancer tends to be rare in men under the age of 40. Although its cause is unknown, a strong family history of the disease, a high-fat diet, being Afro-Caribbean and having little expose to sunlight are all probable risk factors. However, the strongest risk factor of all is simply growing older. Geographically, prostate cancer tends to be more common as you move away from the Equator. It is perhaps significant that Norway and Sweden have the world's highest death rates from this disease, as it is believed that low exposure to sunlight may be an important factor. The symptoms of localised prostate cancer can be very similar to BPH and so it is possible to be lulled into a false sense of security. Symptoms to look out for include:

- A weak urinary stream
- Delay before urinating
- Stop/start urination
- Leaking or dribbling urine
- A frequent need to pass water, especially at night
- A feeling that the bladder never fully empties
- Pain or a burning sensation on passing urine

If prostate cancer is detected early, it can often be cured. At one time the only method of detecting the disease was the digital rectal examination, which, although useful in detecting prostatic enlargement, is in many ways a limited diagnostic tool. Fortunately, this can now be supplemented by the PSA blood test. PSA (prostate specific antigen) is the enzyme and sugar-rich fluid, produced by the prostate, which helps to nourish and carry sperm. In general, the healthier your prostate the lower your PSA count, although this normally rises with age. In a normal prostate gland the cells are healthy and only a very small amount of PSA leaks out into the bloodstream as a result. When prostate cancer develops, more PSA leaks into the bloodstream, which is why measuring PSA in a blood sample can help to diagnose prostate cancer.

However, before we all start jumping for joy at this life-line, it must be stressed that it is not a perfect test. An ideal test for prostate cancer should clearly define men who have cancer and men who do not. Unfortunately, with PSA measurements there can be a grey area as to which patients have BPH and which have prostate cancer. In consequence some men will worry unnecessarily that they have cancer when in fact they do not. On top of this, about half of all men of 80 have prostate cancer, although only 4% will die of it rather than from other causes. The more you look at this cancer the muddier it gets, and PSA results need to be viewed in this context, as 'age-specific' readings. As a general guide, normal PSA ranges are:

Age 40–9: normal PSA result 0–2.5 nanograms/millilitre
50–9: PSA 0–3.5 ng/ml
60–9: PSA 0–4.5 ng/ml
70–9: PSA 0–6.5 ng/ml

To sum up, the advantages of a PSA blood test are:

● It can allow for the early detection of prostate cancer far sooner than would otherwise be available.
● It may allow a doctor to estimate how advanced a prostate cancer may be at the time of diagnosis.
● It may help a doctor predict how well a prostate tumour will respond to certain drugs.
● It can monitor, as a screening tool, men with a strong family history of prostate cancer.
● It is helpful for monitoring how well treatment is progressing.

Then there are the drawbacks:

● There is likely to be needless worry, along with further medical procedures, for some patients who, although they have a positive result, do not have prostate cancer.
● Some men with prostate cancer may have an apparently normal PSA, and although the number is only small the problem remains a major concern.

- A high PSA can't distinguish between an aggressive tumour and a slow-growing one.
- PSA levels can be raised for reasons other than cancer, such as a urine infection or prostatitis.

I must emphasise here that a PSA level which is higher than normal does not necessarily mean you are suffering from prostate cancer. Both prostatitis and BPH can raise the PSA level significantly. However, a raised PSA level means that both a digital rectal examination and a prostate biopsy must follow. A urologist will perform the DRE and subsequently a biopsy will be taken from the prostate via the back passage, usually under a local anaesthetic or mild sedative. The biopsy will indicate whether tumours are present, but again this is not a perfect test, although when combined with ultrasound scanning it can give an assessment of how fast the cancer is growing. If cancer is present, this is graded as one of five stages, ranging from a tiny tumour that may be causing no symptoms to a tumour that has spread to the rest of the body. This grading process is important because treatment options vary accordingly. There are several options, but in the UK the usual treatment is either radical prostatectomy or radiotherapy.

- **Radical prostatectomy.** This is a major surgical proce dure in which the entire prostate gland is removed, usually through a cut in the abdomen. It is performed when the cancer is confined to the prostate gland and requires a hospital stay of ten days or less. Unfortunately, this is not well tolerated in older men or in men with poor health. My view here is that there is a fairly small number of urological surgeons in the UK who are well versed in this procedure as a result of regular practice. This operation is often fiendishly difficult and can have serious side effects. These include a considerable risk of impotence and sexual problems (some studies report that up to 60% of men may suffer from these after the operation), while a small number of men suffer from urinary incontinence after this surgery.

● **Radiotherapy.** This applies X-ray beams to the prostate and surrounding tissues to destroy cancer cells. External beam radiotherapy is the most commonly used method, but another, brachey therapy, is becoming increasingly available. Here tiny radioactive seeds which emit low-level radiation for a year or so are inserted into the cancerous prostate. The effects are localised and tend to affect surrounding structures less than external radiation and also the concentration of radiation to the prostate is probably greater The aim of both of these treatments is to shrink any cancerous cells, and they do offer a potential cure as well as avoiding prolonged catheterisation and surgery.

The treatment is often prolonged, however, and it can be difficult to assess whether treatment has been successful in the short term. Another negative point here is that repeat high-dose radiation treatment must not be given and surgery after radiotherapy carries greater risks and is rarely successful. After you have weighed up the pros and cons with your urologist, the choice between surgery or radiotherapy is ultimately yours. I should add that medical progress means the long-term prospects of patients in both camps are improving all the time.

At best the survival rates with radiotherapy are comparable with those associated with radical prostatectomy, especially if combined with hormone therapy. This aims to treat prostate cancer by depriving the body of the male sex hormone testosterone, on which prostate cancer mostly depends for its growth. This treatment is mainly used to treat cancers which have spread outside the prostate gland or before other treatments such as radiotherapy. Hormone therapy shrinks prostate cancer cells and slows their growth, which in turn can not only reduce symptoms but also make the tumour more receptive to other treatments. Very recent research suggests that hormone patches for women may actually be of benefit in treating prostate cancer in patients with advanced disease. Further research is needed to see if this treatment is free of side effects and does prolong survival, but results so far are encouraging.

In one large Swedish trial recently published in the *New England Journal of Medicine*, men with early prostate cancer were given either radical prostatectomy or a conservative watch-and-wait treatment. After six years 4.6% of the men who had undergone surgery were dead, compared with 9% of those who had received conservative treatment, but, interestingly, the longer-term survival figures were much the same for the two groups.

The old-fashioned adage hammered into medical students remains valid: 'If you don't put your finger in it, you put your foot in it!' Digital rectal examination remains a crucial investigation as abnormal findings here are strongly predictive of prostate cancer. Up to one in eight men with a normal PSA but abnormal findings from a DRE are found to have prostate cancer on biopsy.

Nowadays there is an enormous wealth of readily available information about prostate problems. The internet has allowed information to be disseminated to a unprecedented degree and, as with all health problems, knowledge is power.

There does, though, remain an urgent need to increase awareness of the early symptoms of prostate cancer and to encourage men to seek medical advice sooner than they are doing. This is all the more frustrating because, provided prostate cancer is detected early, treatments are available which offer a good chance of cure.

KEY POINTS

- Prostate enlargement is normal with ageing.
- By the age of 50, 30% of men will have trouble passing urine, but only half of these will consult their doctor.
- It is often difficult to distinguish between symptoms of harmless prostate enlargement and prostate cancer.
- Men in the UK have a 1-in-12 lifetime risk of developing prostate cancer, and this risk is expected to increase dramatically by 2020.
- Prostate cancer is rare in men under 45.
- Normal PSA ranges should be age-specific, in order to be more reliable, and prostate cancer screening remains controversial.
- Treatment options for prostate cancer continue to be the subject of serious debate.

DANGER SIGNS
- Poor urine flow
- Frequent urination during both the day and night
- Blood in the urine
- A feeling of never completely emptying the bladder
- Backache for no obvious reason

6
SEXUAL DIFFICULTIES

'The only time my wife and I had a simultaneous orgasm was when the judge signed the divorce papers.'
– Woody Allen

It will come as no surprise that difficulties with erection are the sexual problem that most commonly troubles middle-aged and older men. Erectile dysfunction, or ED, is certainly what brings at least one or two of them a week to my surgery. I've heard it described as Nature's way of saying 'no hard feelings', but with my medical hat on I suggest a more proper definition: the inability of a man to achieve or maintain an erection sufficient to allow the sexual activity that both he and his partner desire.

My back-of-the-envelope calculations show that at any one time ED affects one in ten men. But, to be more scientific, a very good American study that looked at this problem found that some 52% of men between the ages of 40 and 70 reported some degree of impotence and that this was complete in 10% and moderate in 25% of the sample. We're not talking about a rare occurrence here, but look a man in the eye and ask him if he has sexual problems and he would rather own up to kidnapping the Queen than admit to having difficulties in this area. I can usually tell if a man has come to see me with erection problems because a small patch of carpet about two feet in front of his chair suddenly seems to exert a magnetic fascination for him and his eyes remain fixed on this spot throughout the consultation. This is partly a generational thing. Many older men have not been brought up to discuss such things and, more broadly, the idea is deeply engrained in the psyche of men of all ages that to admit to any kind of difficulty with sexual performance is to admit to failing in their own masculinity. This attitude is understandable, but it's a shame because erectile dysfunction has become a much more openly discussed problem, encouraged by the likes of Pele promoting awareness of it in the worldwide media.

To appreciate why ED is so common, let's first look at what actually triggers and sustains an erection. There are three basic processes at work here. The first is sexual arousal. This should go without saying but you would be surprised at how many men who complain to me about erection problems have no desire for their partner whatsoever. No prizes there for guessing why they have a problem.

Next, sexual desire must be communicated from the brain to the body and allow an increase in the flow of blood to the penis. Finally, blood floods the shaft of the penis. Many men do not realise that the erectile tissue in the penis consists of two blocks of spongy material that become engorged with blood and compress the veins that normally drain blood back out of the organ. As a result the penis expands and becomes rigid. Bingo, an erection.

If something affects any of these processes, ED can result, and so it is clear that the causes of this difficulty can be physical, psychological or both. When I was a medical student most people with such problems were thought by consultants to almost exclusively have a psychological block that was causing their impotence. Many were shuffled off to see counsellors or to have sexual therapy, but it is now known that only about a third of ED cases are due to psychological problems, the rest being due to either physical conditions or – much more frequently, in my opinion – a combination of physical and psychological factors. For example, a minor physical problem that causes an erection to develop more slowly than before may worry the man enough for psychological problems to appear, and so the problem becomes worse. It is probably true to say that in all cases of ED there is, to some degree, a psychological component. Indeed, show me the sexually active man who says he is not worried about impotence and I will show you a liar.

Don't forget that here we are not only talking about problems for the man. ED affects both partners and I've seen many relationships and marriages buckle or break under the strain that it can cause. I remember one 50-year-old man who was bullied by his wife to such an extent about his sexual performance and meeting her sexual demands that total impotence occurred, upon which she gave him an ultimatum to either get an erection or a divorce lawyer. Not surprisingly, such pillow talk failed to have the desired effect and the lawyer got even richer.

PHYSICAL CAUSES OF **ED**

But let's look first at the physical causes of erection problems. Most of these involve the fine system of nerves and blood vessels that serves the penis and the spinal cord. Anything that harms this may affect an erection, and one of the commonest causes here is diabetes. For reasons that are not completely clear, if diabetes control is poor the nerves and fine circulation within the penis can be affected and some studies have said that up to two-thirds of diabetic men eventually report some problem with their erections. However, it's not all bad news as tight diabetic control dramatically reduces this risk, although it can't be completely eliminated. Another problem I often see is that, because the type of diabetes that elderly people tend to develop, Type 2, can have relatively few symptoms in its early stages, by the time diagnosis has occurred and treatment has begun some damage may have been done. So I now make a point of asking potential diabetics whether, as well as the usual symptoms of thirst, tiredness and urinating more often than normal, they are having erection problems.

High blood pressure is another significant risk factor for ED since this predisposes people to develop arteriosclerosis, or hardening of the arteries. This can have the effect of reducing the blood flow to the penis and so cause ED Very often arteriosclerosis is linked to smoking, so, apart from the other health problems it causes, the habit is likely to undermine sexual performance in the long term.

Neurological disorders such as Parkinson's disease and multiple sclerosis, as well as injuries or surgery to the genitals and pelvic area, are all recognised as potential causes of ED. Nor must we forget both alcohol and drug abuse here. Chronic alcohol abuse damages the testes and liver, which in turn lowers the levels of testosterone in the body. This is required by nerves in order to transmit messages from the brain to trigger an erection, and depletion of this chemical is the reason why so many heavy chronic drinkers are impotent. In the short term, too, alcohol can cause problems, because it reduces nerve transmission from the penis to the brain, which is why Shakespeare said it 'promotes desire but takes away performance'.

Doctors themselves can be guilty of causing erection problems in their patients by their prescribing habits. Some medicines used to treat high blood pressure, such as diuretics and beta-blockers, are generally acknowledged as possible causes of ED. Some antidepressant and anti-psychotic drugs also have this effect. Many men seem to accept that their medication has a damping effect on their erection and so do not mention it to their doctor. This is a shame as there may be a suitable alternative drug which does not have this side effect.

PSYCHOLOGICAL CAUSES OF ED

'Performance anxiety' is a common cause of temporary ED and most men at some point in their life experience it. This is usually nothing to worry about, but if it occurs it is vital to assume that you do not have a problem, otherwise you can expect to fail the next time. Over the age of 50 it is also important to remember that it is quite normal for sexual performance to change. It may take longer for erections to develop, these may not be as hard as before and orgasms may be less intense. Ejaculation volume is usually reduced and recovery time between erections increases, but all these are normal effects of ageing.

I'm still not sure whether I was being wound up or not, but I remember an 87-year-old man coming to see me looking depressed, sitting down and saying, 'Doc, I think I'm impotent.' I gave him my standard speech about how, as the body ages, its functions slow down, explaining that it is completely normal to suffer some decrease in sexual desire and that worrying about this would normally make things worse. I then asked him when he began to think he was impotent, and I took some time to recover my composure when he told me it was twice the day before and again that morning. Roll on, 87.

Other psychological causes include depression, relationship problems or the partner's lack of interest in sex. It's also a fact that many men experiencing ED try to hide the problem from their partner by avoiding sex, which only makes it worse. Common ruses that men use include claiming to have a headache or be exhausted at bedtime (usually because they are having to work harder than usual), staying up late to make sure their partner is asleep by the time they get to bed or going to bed early so that they are asleep before their partner joins them.

Another important thing to remember is that sexual function is influenced by a person's general well-being. ED may simply be a sign that not enough attention is being paid to maintaining a healthy lifestyle. Even the most effective treatments for ED can't be expected to work against a background of poor sleep, constant fatigue and inadequate diet. Poor relationships are also a big factor here. If you and your partner are not talking to each other out of the bedroom, then your performance in it is unlikely to be much good either.

Whether the causes are physical, psychological or a combination of the two, it is safe to say, given the number of surveys that are being done on ED, that this is a very common problem. It is clear also that it is often under-reported, under-diagnosed and under-treated. Many men choose not to report the problem to their doctor because they feel that somehow it is not a proper medical condition, but most of those who do are hugely relieved when they are reassured that it is and told that it can be treated.

Men, both young and old, are now looking for a quick fix for erection problems. While this is often not possible, the efficacy of modern treatments is now such that a man can often continue a satisfactory sexual relationship against the odds, whereas once he would have had no chance of doing so. Most doctors will first try the so-called 'physical' treatments and then consider a psychological approach if these fail. There are three main kinds of physical treatment to look at here: drugs, mechanical aids and surgery.

DRUG TREATMENT

This is perhaps the commonest way of treating ED in the developed world, and although Viagra (Sildenafil) opened the floodgates, it is only one of a number of drugs now available that can be taken orally to treat erectile dysfunction. Viagra works directly on the tissues of the penis to increase the blood flow to it and so cause an erection. The drug can have mild side effects, such as causing blue vision or sweating, but, more importantly, it should be used with care by men with cardiac complaints. I must have heard every Viagra joke there is, but I still remember with a smile being told, in all seriousness, by a 60-year-old that a consignment of Viagra had been hijacked near his home and the police were looking for a bunch of hardened criminals.

A number of alternatives to Viagra are now on the market. Apomorphine (Uprima) works within the brain rather than directly on the penile tissue to increase nerve signals to the penis which result in an erection. Some men find this drug works more quickly than Viagra. Tadalafil (Cialis), which works in a similar manner to Viagra, represents the next generation of treatment and is said to have fewer side effects in some men, as well as having the potential to work slightly faster.

We are now starting to see 'me-too' medicines, which are basically variations on the same theme. The most recent oral treatment for ED launched in the UK is Vardenafil (Levetra). So wide is the choice now that doctors are almost at the point where we have to say, you pay your money and you take your choice.

Slightly less popular drug treatments are injections of Alprostadil. This again works directly on the penis to increase and maintain blood flow in it, but it works in a slightly different way to Viagra. It can either be injected directly into the penis (which is less painful than you might imagine) or inserted as a pellet directly into the urethral channel of the penis and, again, this is not particularly uncomfortable.

MECHANICAL AIDS

The steady increase in the number of drug therapies for erectile dysfunction means that mechanical aids have somewhat fallen out of favour, and I, for one, can understand why. Perhaps the simplest of these is known as the constriction ring, which is a rubber or silicone ring designed to sit firmly around the base of the penis. It is tight enough to reduce or stop blood flowing out of the penis through the penile veins but not so tight that it stops blood coming into the penis through the arteries, which are at a higher pressure than the veins. The consequent build-up of pressure means that blood flow increases within the penis and there is an improvement in the quality of the erection. This method can be effective once there is an erection but the results can be disappointing if this has not been achieved.

Another previously popular mechanical aid is the vacuum pump, which has been around for decades and looks rather a Heath Robinson affair. This is essentially a plastic chamber which is placed over the penis. Air is extracted from the chamber by means of a pump, since creating a partial vacuum around the penis allows blood to be drawn into it more effectively. If a sustainable erection is achieved, a constriction ring can be placed around the base of the penis to help maintain it. The device can be surprisingly effective and success rates of up to 90% have been reported. My experience of couples who use such aids is that if they have been tried readily as an initial option they can be very effective, but if they are used as a last resort couples are often dissatisfied. With both the constriction ring and the vacuum pump, there are no side effects (although there can be scrotal bruising on occasion), but some men complain that their sensation is affected when using a constriction ring, and some partners have told me that the penis feels colder than normal. Even so, such simple devices should not be discounted, especially by couples who prefer not to try drug treatment.

With the increase in male cosmetic surgery extending into penile elongation and thickening, surgical techniques involving the penis develop all the time, so it is not surprising that methods to treat erectile dysfunction are now available. In my view these should be resorted to only when all else has failed, and even then with great caution. I do accept, though, that in cases where the surgeon is vastly experienced, there is a high degree of patient satisfaction with these procedures. Whatever the technique used, the basic method is to insert rods into the shaft of the penis under the skin. These are known as penile prostheses – imagine high-tech pipe cleaners and you will not be far off the mark. They can be bent up and down at will but their insertion destroys erectile tissue inside the penis and after this operation no form of drug therapy for the original problem is effective.

A slightly more sophisticated variation is a fluid-filled prosthesis which can be pumped up as required. However, this needs both tubing and a fluid reservoir inserted either within the scrotum or lower abdomen – not something you can nip in to have done in your lunch hour.

When I was a medical student it was the vogue among some enthusiastic surgeons to tie off the veins in the penis with the aim of reducing blood flow out of the organ and so improve erection quality. In some men this did have dramatically effective results, but almost always this success withered after a year or so, with the result that this method has largely been abandoned.

PSYCHOLOGICAL TREATMENTS

An important thing to bear in mind about the success of drugs such as Viagra is that they may well cure the symptoms and yet they do nothing about the cause of the problem. Undeniably, they can make erection possible once more, but if there is an underlying psychological difficulty this will not have been addressed. It is because of this that ED should never be viewed as a male problem in isolation and should always involve the couple if possible. I should say, though, that there are many women who choose not to visit my surgery with their partners, instead leaving them to come home with the magic pill in the hope that all will be well again. Some of them are subsequently disappointed, as they did not realise that because of the NHS's limited drugs budget the government has ruled that only certain patients can receive ED treatment on the NHS.

There are three main groups which fall into this category. Firstly, there are men with the following conditions: prostate cancer, diabetes, multiple sclerosis, Parkinson's disease, polio, spina bifida, kidney failure, spinal cord injuries or severe pelvic injuries, single gene urological disease, and those who have had prostate or radical pelvic surgery. Secondly, there are men who are severely distressed as a result of their impotence. To my mind this is a huge grey area and some men do exploit this definition. Finally, there are men who are diagnosed as suffering from impotence or who were receiving treatment on the NHS on or before 14 September 1998.

Sex therapists and counsellors can be very effective in helping couples work through psychological and sexual issues but, like cognitive behavioural therapists to treat depression, they are as rare as hen's teeth in the NHS. Most need to be seen privately and the ones who are under the auspices of the NHS are swamped with work. Despite this, it is always sensible to discuss the possibility of seeing a sex therapist with your doctor as this approach may provide far more long-term benefit than either drug treatment or mechanical aids.

OTHER SEXUAL DIFFICULTIES

Men have other sexual problems besides ED, of course, and the ones I'm most often asked about are loss of sexual desire and problems with ejaculation.

● **Loss of sexual desire.** This mean a lack interest in sex which causes sufficient concern to the man and/or his partner for it to be seen as a problem by the couple. The main symptom here tends to be that you rarely (or never) feel like having sex, or if you do feel like it at times, it's far less often than your partner does. The condition is far more common than usually realised and in a recent large survey some 15% of men of between 18 and 59 claimed to lack interest in sex. It is possible that you may simply have a naturally lower level of sexual desire than your partner, and here the main problem is negotiating some sort of compromise. There are various other causes, most of which are psychological, such as relationship difficulties, sexual boredom (some serial monogamists say that the best aphrodisiac is a change of partner), depression, mental exhaustion and stress. Tried-and-tested first steps include trying to improve the quality of your sleep, cope better with stress and sort out any relationship problems, and finding ways of spicing up your sex life, such as using different positions and trying new times and places.

If you feel you may be depressed, seek help at once, because if this is the case you may kiss a good sex life goodbye for ever. Lack of sexual appetite is one of the curses of depression. Try regular exercise as a way of lifting your mood and with it your sexual desire for your partner.

You should certainly see a doctor if, despite all you do to boost it, your low level of sexual desire persists and is causing problems in a relationship. If you also have other symptoms, such as exhaustion, a reduction in facial hair growth or a loss of body hair, shrinking testicles or muscle weakness, ask whether these could all be signs of testosterone deficiency.

The main treatments for most people here are sexual counselling and, in a very small number of cases, testosterone supplements. But what may also help greatly is simply talking to your partner about your feelings and finding ways of developing closeness that are not exclusively linked to sex.

Whatever you do, avoid cranky-sounding cures and 'miracle' remedies on the internet, including so-called aphrodisiacs such as oysters or ginseng. If there were evidence that any of these works we'd most likely know about it already.

● **Premature (rapid) ejaculation.** This is where ejaculation occurs more quickly than a man and his partner would wish. It can be a very destructive problem in a relationship, often causing mounting frustration and bitterness, however close the couple. The usual problem men discuss with me here is that they climax as soon as they penetrate or if not then, very soon afterwards. Many men do not realise that this is the commonest sexual problem affecting them, with about one in three men of all ages suffering from it. Rarely is it caused by a physical problem. Among the most frequent causes are anxiety about sex (often owing to a fear of causing pregnancy, guilt or performance-related stress), relationship difficulties and the lasting effects of teenage sexual experiences or childhood abuse.

Unfortunately, solving this problem can be tricky since what you need to do above all is find better ways of coping with stress and resolve any personal or relationship difficulties you may have with your partner. I tend to see men in my surgery with this difficulty when it has become persistent and is causing a good deal of anxiety. There is often little I'm able to do that has an immediate effect, so specialist clinics and qualified sex therapists are usually a first-line treatment here.

Sex therapy has two main techniques that form the

backbone of any treatment. The first is the 'stop-start technique', where you or your partner masturbates you until you are near the point of ejaculation. You then stop immediately, however quickly this has happened, and rest for 30–60 seconds before starting again. This process is repeated half a dozen times or so during each session. The second method is the 'squeeze technique'. Again your penis is stimulated until you are near the point of ejaculation, but instead of stopping, this time you or your partner firmly squeezes around your penis just below the glans (head). This has the effect of preventing ejaculation, provided you have not already got too close to climaxing to avoid it.

The point of both these techniques is that, over time, you can begin to recognise what it feels like to be near the moment when you can't stop yourself coming. If you are able to do that during sex itself, you can then slow down or stop until the feeling fades. Once a man knows he can control his ejaculation in this way, his confidence increases and eventually the whole process occurs without his being aware of it.

I'm not keen on using drugs for this problem but do occasionally prescribe a local anaesthetic gel that can be applied to the penis to reduce its sensitivity. This is by no means a perfect solution to the problem as it works in some men but not every time, it doesn't help others at all, some men are allergic to it and the gel may be transferred to your partner during intercourse and cause a loss of sexual sensitivity in them.

Many antidepressant drugs have the side effect of reducing sex drive and slowing down progress towards ejaculation, but these are powerful tablets, they may not work well anyway and can have other unpleasant side effects.

Simpler methods are to masturbate frequently, which will often delay subsequent ejaculations, and to wear a condom to reduce penile sensitivity.

We all know the classical Australian foreplay line, 'Brace yourself, Sheila', but instead of going down this manly path, try not focusing on penetration during sex. You can often reduce the pressure on yourself if you don't attempt penetration until your partner has already had an orgasm. Talking to your partner about your problem can also help to relieve sexual anxiety. Relaxation exercises are very effective in delaying ejaculation, although men often dismiss them as too 'feminine', which is a pity since they can be easily performed. A classic example is to tense and relax each of your muscle groups in turn, starting with your feet and then moving up your body. Clench each set of muscles for a few seconds, focus on the feeling and then gradually relax, working steadily up the body to finish with your forehead. As a way of reducing the muscle tension which stress causes, including in the genitals, it can be hard to beat.

Provided they have determination, persistence and an understanding partner, many men find it quite possible to develop good ejaculatory control.

● **Retarded (delayed) ejaculation.** This is the inability to ejaculate, or being able to do so only after a very long delay. About 5% of men are affected by this problem, and in the majority the cause is psychological. Performance anxiety, self-consciousness about their body, a belief that sex is somehow dirty or immoral, and stress or relationship difficulties can all lead to retarded ejaculation. Many men with this problem tell me they can ejaculate normally when they masturbate alone, but are totally unable to come when inside their partner. This does not necessarily mean that there is not enough stimulation to the penis – there always is – but confirms that the problem is psychological. As suggested earlier, talking openly with a sympathetic partner about your difficulty can play an important role here.

It is also common for men around the age of 70 to experience failure of ejaculation as a normal part of the ageing process. One aspect of this is decreased penile sensitivity, which means older men need more prolonged and direct penile stimulation to achieve ejaculation than younger men. Sometimes ejaculation fails just because they do not have sufficient penile stimulation. It may also be that the side effects of certain antidepressant drugs are responsible, in which case ask your doctor if it is possible to replace any drug that might be implicated. Alternatively, the problem may arise from nerve damage caused by pelvic injury, surgery or diabetes.

Whatever your age, you should see your GP if your problem persists and is causing you anxiety or affecting your relationship. If these are not relevant, I usually advise about self-help measures or refer the patient to a specialist clinic or qualified sex therapist. 'Superstimulation', such as using a vibrator or body oil combined with vigorous rubbing, can help, as can the drug yohimbine, although this can have side effects and men with high blood pressure should not take it. Always avoid penetration until you are very near the point of ejaculation. Finally, as with premature ejaculation, relaxation exercises are always worth trying.

Woody Allen may have said, 'Don't knock masturbation – it's sex with someone you love', but for most men common sense, allied to honesty and patience, reaps rewards in the end.

KEY POINTS

- Male sexual problems are far more common than most people realise.
- Over half of all men over 40 experience problems to some degree.
- The causes of sexual difficulties can be either physical, psychological or both.
- Usually the most difficult thing for a man to do is take the first step of admitting he has a problem.
- Many cases require patience and understanding rather than formal treatment.
- A variety of methods, including mechanical devices, drugs and, less commonly, sex therapy and psychological counselling, are used to treat erectile dysfunction and other sexual difficulties.

7

BOWEL PROBLEMS

GP: *What did you operate on Mr Smith for?*
Surgeon: *A hundred pounds.*
GP: *No, I mean what did he have?*
Surgeon: *A hundred pounds.*
— **19th-century *Punch* cartoon**

I've often said that the Americans have their cholesterol, the French their liver and the British — well, the British have their bowels. This attachment is seen not just in our predilection for toilet humour. As long as I enquire politely of patients how their bowels have been, they usually feel satisfied that they have had a good consultation, whatever else I may have said. Despite our concern for our bowels, a survey published by Cancer Research UK found that over half of us never checked to see if they had been bleeding before flushing the loo, while not even one in four people recognised the symptoms of bowel cancer.

BOWEL CANCER

As well as being the second biggest cause of cancer death in the UK, bowel cancer is the third commonest of all the forms of the disease. Frustratingly, it is also one of the most readily treated if detected early enough, with some 90% of early cancers of the bowel being curable. Every year there are some 30,000 new cases and 17,000 people die from it, with 95% of cases occurring in the over-50s and the disease being more common in men.

There is a strong genetic element to this particular cancer, also called colorectal cancer, and some 6–7% of people with it have a family history of the disease. If you have a close relative, such as a parent or sibling, who has been diagnosed with bowel cancer before the age of 45, you yourself have a fourfold increased risk of developing it. However, this risk is age-related, so if the relative is diagnosed with bowel cancer after the age of 60, your risk is the same as the rest of the general population.

Aside from genetics, our Western diet undoubtedly is the main player here. A typical low-fibre, high-fat diet is believed to account for 80% of cases of bowel cancer in the developed world, and this is why it is such a preventable disease.

Other risk factors include an unhealthy, inactive lifestyle, or the existence of other bowel disorders, such as ulcerative colitis or Crohn's disease, which cause chronic inflammation of the bowel lining.

The main symptoms of bowel cancer are:

- A change in bowel habit, such as bouts of constipation or diarrhoea, lasting more than two weeks
- Rectal bleeding. Here there is either blood mixed in with the motions or the motions are very dark. It is wrong to assume that if rectal bleeding is bright red it must always be from piles since, depending on where the cancer is, that blood can be bright red too
- Abdominal pain or pain on opening the bowels
- Weight loss

- Poor appetite
- Tiredness
- A feeling of never emptying the bowels fully, or of wanting to go to the toilet again when you have just been

There are a number of harmless conditions which can cause similar symptoms, so if you have some of these it does not mean you have bowel cancer. It simply means you need to get checked out. At present there is no automatic or generalised bowel-screening programme for bowel cancer in people without symptoms, but you should certainly be examined if you have any of the above symptoms or if the disease runs in your family. Your doctor will take a general history, examine you abdominally, do a rectal examination with the finger and, if appropriate, refer you to a specialist for further tests. They may also examine a sample of your motions for blood, but this should not be used by itself as harmless conditions can cause a positive result here.

If bowel cancer is present, the chances of it being cured are very good, provided it is caught early enough. The caveat here, of course, is those last few words. Eight out of ten people with bowel cancer have surgery, but in half of these the cancer recurs because it has spread to other organs, especially the liver. Fifty per cent of the people who have had surgery live for at least three years and 40% are alive at least ten years later.

Trials are currently in progress to assess whether a single flexible sigmoidoscopy examination at the age of 60 could be a safe and cost-effective way of cutting the number of deaths from bowel cancer. Early figures show that about one in three hundred people screened had undiagnosed bowel cancer. The procedure uses a flexible fibre-optic telescope to examine the large bowel for small growths or polyps, which are often the early signs of this cancer. Because these often grow slowly and painlessly, an increased awareness of the symptoms to look out for is vital. So, if your bowel habits have changed, you have blood in your motions or you have any other worrying symptoms, see your doctor straight away.

Polyps have the potential to become cancerous, although most prove not to be, and these can be removed surgically during endoscopic examination. If the cancer has not spread or is localised within a polyp, its removal is the end of the story and long-term screening then takes place. Unfortunately, at diagnosis most cancers are found in the gut wall and so require surgical removal followed by a course of chemotherapy. Treatment in the form of X-rays or radio-therapy before surgery also reduces the chances of bowel cancer returning and, depending on where the cancer is, various operations can be performed. It may be necessary to have surgery in which the cut end of the large bowel is brought to the surface of the skin so that in future the motions empty into a bag attached to the front of the abdomen. This is called a colostomy or ileostomy, according to which part of the bowel is used.

To give yourself the best chance of defending against this common cancer, you should act on the following points:

- Eat a diet low in fat and rich in fruit and vegetables.
- Cut down on tea and coffee.
- Eat plenty of high-fibre cereals, pasta and wholemeal bread.
- Keep your intake of red meat to a minimum, as well as cutting back on fried foods, sweets, chocolates and cakes. Trim the fat off meat and poultry.

- Stay as trim as you can, as obesity is a risk factor here.
- Try to stay active, even if this is as simple as walking briskly every day, because people who exercise throughout their lives run the lowest risk of this form of cancer.
- Get to know your bowel habits and what is normal for you. If these change, let your doctor know. Check your stools for signs of blood before flushing the loo.
- Do not rely solely on home testing kits because these can give false positive results when certain foods, such as beetroot, have been eaten.
- Remember the golden mantra – if in doubt, get checked out.

CONSTIPATION

There is a huge amount of confusion about what a normal bowel habit is. Many people swear blind that if someone is not opening their bowels every day then there is something terribly wrong, whereas the normal range of bowel movements varies from three times a day to three times a week. In fact, research suggests that so-called normal bowel function – going to the toilet once a day – occurs in only half the adult population. As far as constipation is concerned, you can be said to have the condition if you have to strain to pass your stools and these are hard and difficult to pass, and if you are opening your bowels less than three times a week

Constipated people also often report that they feel tired, sluggish and bloated and have generalised low abdominal discomfort. Up to 40% of people strain when they open their bowels and 1% of British people consult their doctor every year about this problem alone. It has been estimated that up to 14 million may be technically defined as suffering from constipation. There are many common causes for this, including a diet containing insufficient fibre and, more importantly here, insufficient fluid. Most of us are dehydrated and because the large intestine absorbs water from the food passing through it, by the time you are ready to open your bowels most of the water will have been absorbed. If there is not enough fluid in the body to start with, the stools become hard and dry and are therefore difficult to pass.

Many people also ignore the urge to go to the toilet, either because they are too busy or think they will put it off until later. I well remember an eminent professor at St Bartholomew's Hospital gravely telling me, during a ward round, that the secret of a healthy bowel was 'never to ignore calls to stool, my boy'. Other common causes of constipation include medicines such as iron supplements, antacids containing aluminium, antidepressants and narcotics, while taking too many laxatives can have a rebound effect by making the bowel work both less and more sluggishly, worsening constipation. Emotional upsets can be a cause, as can a lack of exercise and medical conditions such as an underactive thyroid gland, haemorrhoids, irritable bowel syndrome and damage to the nerves of the spinal cord. Tumours and serious bowel inflammation can cause both constipation and diarrhoea.

To try to prevent constipation, drink at least eight glasses of water a day and cut down on the amount of tea and coffee you drink as these can dehydrate you. Don't ignore the urge to pass motions and set aside time after breakfast or meals to do so undisturbed. Remember to eat a diet that is well balanced and full of fresh fruit, vegetables and fibre. It is best not to use laxatives long term, but if you find that you have been using these for more than three to four weeks, consult your doctor. Certainly you should see your doctor immediately if your stools contain blood or if there is a change in your bowel pattern lasting more than a couple of weeks. Most cases of simple constipation clear up when more fibre and fluid are added to the diet, but if necessary these may be supplemented with fibre sachets or stool softeners.

DIARRHOEA

When the stools are too loose or too frequent, the problem is most often diarrhoea. This can be acute, which means it occurs suddenly and lasts a few days, or chronic, when it can last more than three weeks. Nasty stomach pains, chills and fever and occasionally vomiting usually accompany acute diarrhoea. Virtually everyone has a bout of it at least once in their life. One of my most vivid student memories, which I've long tried to blank out from my brain, is of the consequences of eating a week-old beefburger that I found in a fridge and was too lazy to throw out. Ever since then I've had a very healthy respect for food poisoning.

Common causes of acute diarrhoea include things like my good friend that ancient beefburger, undercooked meat or eggs and poor personal hygiene. Alcohol, especially beer, is well known for this, as is travel in various parts of the world, and taking antibiotics, which can alter the normal balance of bacteria in the gut. Anxiety is another typical cause, with about 20% of people suffering from what is known as performance-anxiety diarrhoea at some time. Good examples here are the best man who is worried about giving his speech and the student facing an exam.

Chronic diarrhoea, by contrast, often has other causes. These include a constitutional intolerance to dairy products or wheat, a poor diet and generalised bowel conditions such as irritable bowel syndrome and inflammatory bowel disease. Pancreatic problems and an overactive thyroid gland can also trigger long-term diarrhoea, as can bowel cancer and diabetes and its treatment.

As most cases of diarrhoea clear up after a few days there is no need to see your doctor, but if you report that it has continued longer than this, a laboratory examination of a stool sample may need to be arranged. Always wash your hands thoroughly after going to the lavatory, don't drink alcohol if you have diarrhoea and take sensible precautions such as drinking bottled water instead of tap water when travelling abroad. During acute diarrhoea drink plenty of fluids or rehydration solutions to replenish any salts you may have lost from the body. If you are on a business trip or holiday, it makes sense to take anti-diarrhoeal drugs such as loperamide to tide you over until you return home. These can also be taken long term in the less common situation of having a generally overactive bowel and a tendency towards diarrhoea, but this should be the exception rather than the rule.

INFLAMMATORY BOWEL DISEASE

When I talk about inflammatory bowel disease (IBD) I mean something very different from irritable bowel syndrome, which I deal with below. IBD is an umbrella name for Crohn's disease and ulcerative colitis (UC). Crohn's disease is an inflammatory illness which can affect any part of the bowel, from the mouth to the anus, although it usually involves the small intestine. The whole of the bowel wall is targeted rather than just the lining and this causes severe inflammation and swelling of the affected area. In ulcerative colitis it is the lining of the large bowel that becomes inflamed and here tiny ulcers develop which can bleed. UC does not affect the small bowel and can affect the rectum only, in which case it is called proctitis.

Over 120,000 people in Britain have IBD and there are over 8,000 new cases each year. Six out of ten sufferers are under 30, but it can occur at any age. No one knows exactly why they should develop it in the first place but about a fifth of people with Crohn's disease have a relative with some form of IBD. Infection has also been proposed as a cause but the case is not proven. Stress does not cause IBD but severe anxiety, viral illness and antibiotics can all trigger attacks in someone who is known to have the condition. Crohn's disease and UC are not infectious and not cancerous, but if either significantly affects the large bowel for many years, then the risk of bowel cancer does progressively increase. Because no one knows exactly why they occur, it is difficult to prevent these diseases.

The most common symptoms of Crohn's disease are:

- Low abdominal pain
- Diarrhoea and bleeding
- Weight loss
- Vomiting, nausea and occasionally fever
- Anaemia with tiredness
- Painful joints and sore, red eyes owing to inflammation of the eye muscle
- Painful red swellings on the legs and mouth ulcers

In ulcerative colitis the greater the extent of the disease the more severe the symptoms. In proctitis, where only the rectum is affected, symptoms are milder and usually include diarrhoea, discomfort and bleeding, but in UC in which the entire gut is inflamed severe symptoms are similar to those of Crohn's disease. Acute attacks usually cause diarrhoea with blood and mucus, there may be fever and lethargy and there may also be a profound anaemia with paleness and tiredness.

Specialist treatment is usually warranted, not only to achieve a correct diagnosis but also to maintain remission and allow as normal a lifestyle as possible. Drugs certainly control the symptoms and with Crohn's disease anti-inflammatories such as steroids damp down the inflammation of the bowel. Anti-diarrhoeal drugs and painkillers may also be used, as in ulcerative colitis, where treatment depends on how severe it is.

Steroids are a popular choice, as are drugs such as Azathioprine, which is taken long term to reduce inflammation of the bowel lining. In very severe cases of IBD surgery may be necessary. This may sound dramatic, but for people who have struggled for years with their symptoms this can come as a relief.

Trying to prevent IBD occurring is almost impossible, but in general terms try to avoid any foods such as spices or alcohol which make symptoms worse. If you feel there are certain foods that trigger symptoms, you may want to try an exclusion diet to see if this helps. Complementary therapy such as meditation or yoga may be used to ease stress and foster the positive mental outlook that is very important in dealing with this condition.

HAEMORRHOIDS (PILES)

Almost every man suffers from piles at some time in his life, but you will not hear many of them talking about it in the pub. Haemorrhoids, as piles are properly called, are swollen blood vessels in and around the rectum, and they can be either internal or external. An internal pile may squeeze outside the back passage when you open your bowels and this may be painful or tender but can be pushed back inside. Occasionally one remains and the muscles around the rectum squeeze it so tightly that the blood in the pile clots and becomes hard and painful. This is known as a strangulated haemorrhoid, and although it is not dangerous, it certainly brings tears to the eyes.

By the age of 50 at least half the general population are regularly suffering from piles. Anything that puts a strain on the abdomen can trigger the condition. Most men over the age of 50 develop them as a result of prolonged straining to open their bowels, which puts constant pressure on the veins around the back passage. Men are also more prone to develop them from lifting heavy weights, having a persistent cough or being overweight. However, the old wives' tale about getting piles from sitting on a cold surface is simply not true. If you have piles already, this may make them worse, but it won't cause them in the first place.

A common sign of piles is bright red blood on the toilet paper and sometimes in the toilet bowl. A little blood looks a lot here, with the result that many men believe they are bleeding to death even though they have passed no more than a tablespoon or so. There can be a feeling of a lump at the anus, often accompanied by itching, and there can be quite severe pain in that area. However, some people have no symptoms at all or only occasional symptoms. The main treatments are creams and suppositories, available over the counter rather than from your doctor, which help the itching and discomfort. A short bath in warm water is also soothing, as is a cold compress or ice pack used to reduce swelling.

To try to prevent piles in the first place, always go to the lavatory when you get the urge and keep your stools soft by eating fibre and drinking plenty of water, herbal drinks or fruit juices.

If your piles don't clear up in a couple of weeks or become painful, it is best to see your doctor. You should certainly do so at once if you have rectal bleeding. Haemorrhoids sometimes need to be dealt with surgically, and most of the procedures are now done as either a day case or in an outpatient clinic. These minor operations include ligation, in which a small rubber band is placed around the haemorrhoids to cut off their blood supply, which makes them wither away in a few days. Ligation has a good success rate, although the piles may return in the future. Another treatment is injection sclerotherapy, in which a chemical solution is injected around the piles to shrink them. In the most severe cases a formal haemorrhoidectomy under a general anaesthetic is used to remove them.

Piles never become cancerous and are a nuisance that has to be lived with rather than a serious medical condition. However, always make sure that your symptoms are due to piles rather than simply assuming this is the problem.

IRRITABLE BOWEL SYNDROME

This is the name given to a range of symptoms which affect the digestive system. IBS is a diagnosis of exclusion, which means that usually it is made after other possibilities have been ruled out. It is the commonest gastroenterological disorder of all, affecting at least half of all patients attending gastroenterology outpatient clinics and probably one in five people worldwide. It is not hereditary or due to food allergy or bowel inflammation and there may be a number of other symptoms not related to the gut. The problem may occur at any age but often peaks in a person's early twenties and again after the age of 40, with men and women being equally affected.

The cause of IBS remains unclear but is probably due to a combination of factors, all of which contribute to an increased sensitivity of the bowel, which in turn leads to bowel spasm. As a disruption of the bowel's normal workings rather than a serious disease, it is sometimes called 'functional' bowel disorder.

The symptoms vary from person to person, but all patients tend to have at least some of the following:

● Abdominal pain. Usually colicky, and often the main problem. This may be felt anywhere but especially on the lower left side of the abdomen. Opening the bowels or passing wind may relieve the pain.
● A feeling of fullness and abdominal bloating. Clothes may feel gradually tighter through the day as the bloating often worsens with the passage of time. There may also be rumbling bowel sounds and wind.
● Diarrhoea and constipation. There may be an alternating pattern of bowel movements in which loose motions are passed several times a day and then, some days later, hard, pellet-like stools that are difficult to pass. On opening the bowels, discomfort or a sensation of not fully

emptying them may be felt. Bleeding from the back passage is never a sign of IBS; nor is significant weight loss.

● Other symptoms include tiredness, backache and urinary problems.

With patients that may have IBS I perform tests primarily to exclude any other more serious bowel disorders, some of which can mimic it. In younger patients simple blood tests such as a full blood count and tests looking for any inflammation in the body may be enough to confirm the harmless nature of the symptoms. In older people X-rays of the bowel (a barium enema) or colonoscopy (an examination of the bowel using a flexible fibre-optic telescope) may need to be done to rule out inflammation, polyps or tumours. Any more worrying symptoms, such as weight loss or blood in the motions, warrant a full investigation, usually by a hospital specialist. Occasionally the problem's response to a trial of IBS treatment may help to establish the diagnosis.

Although symptoms of IBS can be very troublesome, they do not cause serious complications and usually settle with time and little treatment. Understanding the diagnosis and knowing there is nothing seriously wrong often helps sufferers considerably. Simple advice on diet and eating habits is also important, as is a recognition of how stress usually makes symptoms worse.

The specific symptoms of IBS and common treatments for them are:

● Pain. Many people find peppermint oil helpful. Prescribed anti-spasmodic tablets are also often effective; these can be taken either regularly or when the pain occurs.

- Constipation. Increasing both the amount of fluid drunk daily and the amount of fibre in the diet is helpful here, although initially some people may find an increase in fibre makes their symptoms, especially bloating, worse. Occasionally additional laxative treatment may be needed, but stimulant laxatives should be avoided or used very sparingly.
- Diarrhoea. Loperamide, which acts by drying out the motions, is usually used intermittently. In severe cases codeine can be used, but side effects such as nausea and drowsiness are more common with this.
- Bloating and wind. This is often very difficult to treat, but when it is linked to constipation, as it often is, treating this condition helps the problem. A prokinetic agent, which regulates normal bowel activity, is effective in a small number of cases.
- If severe stress, anxiety or depression seem to be causing all the symptoms, treatment with a simple low-dose anti-depressant is often helpful.

Most people with IBS have either self-limiting episodes of symptoms, or repeated attacks, often linked to stressful events. IBS *never* turns into other, more serious bowel problems such as cancer or colitis. Fortunately, there is a great deal you can do to help yourself here. A well-balanced, healthy diet, eaten little and often, usually reduces symptoms, as does avoiding rich, fatty or spicy foods. There is no specific 'anti-IBS' diet, as foods which make one sufferer's symptoms worse will not affect someone else. Dairy products, bread and cereals are all often linked to symptoms, but IBS is not a food allergy. Drinking at least eight glasses of water each day may also help and is anyway a healthy habit.

KEY POINTS

- Bowel problems are extremely common in both men and women over 50.
- Many cases are minor, but with increasing age the risk of conditions such as bowel cancer grows.
- Never ignore any unusual bowel symptoms – always have them checked out.
- It is a myth that you have to open your bowels once a day for good health.
- A diet rich in fibre and fresh fruit and vegetables, allied to a high fluid intake, is a bowel-friendly one.

DANGER SIGNS

- Any change in your normal bowel habit lasting more than two weeks
- Weight loss
- Abdominal pain or bloating
- A feeling of never properly emptying your bowels, or of needing to open them again soon after doing so
- Bleeding from the rectum
- Passing blood or mucus in the motions

8
JOINTS AND BONES

'Orthodox medicine has not, unfortunately, managed to find an answer to your complaint. Luckily, however, for you, I happen to be a quack.'
– Overheard in a doctor's surgery

Several times a week one patient or another shuffles up to me holding one of their joints and says something like, 'My screws are bad today, Doc', 'It's me arthritis' or 'I'm stiff as a board.' What they are referring to is varying degrees of arthritis, a disease in which the joints of the body become inflamed. This is such a common problem that most of us will suffer from it to some extent at some time in our lives and at least 15% of the population of the UK have, at any one time, a significant problem with either arthritis or arthritis-linked conditions. People are often shocked to learn that there are over 200 different types of arthritis, which vary hugely in how fast or slowly they develop and how destructive they can be. By far the commonest is osteoarthritis, sometimes known as wear-and-tear arthritis. This is followed by rheumatoid arthritis, believed to affect nearly 1% of the world's population. In general, the longer we live the more likely we are to develop arthritis, but in addition to age other factors are implicated. These include excessive joint use (as seen in the many ex-professional footballers in their forties with ankle and knee arthritis), stress, injury, viral infections and problems of the immune system.

ARTHRITIS

Many GPs tend to talk only about osteoarthritis and rheumatoid arthritis, but there are five basic groups that form the bulk of my arthritis workload and it's worth looking at these individually:

● **Wear-and-tear arthritis.** In this condition, also known as osteoarthritis or degenerative disease, the protective cartilage on the ends of bones progressively wears away, leaving bone rubbing on bone. It is as if your joint's shock absorber has worn out and this causes stiffness, pain and difficulty in moving the joint.

● **Synovial membrane inflammation.** This is the rheumatoid arthritis group, where the synovial membrane, which is on the outside of each joint and produces joint lubrication, becomes inflamed. It causes the whole of the joint to swell up and become red and warm. If this inflammation is allowed to progress unchecked, serious destruction of the joint will occur.

● **Ligament and tendon inflammation.** In such cases of arthritis the inflammation is not actually in or around the synovial membrane of the joint but slightly outside it or where the ligaments and tendons go into the bones. This is the third commonest type of arthritis, after osteoarthritis and rheumatoid arthritis, and can affect up to one in 200 people. Of the problems in this group, perhaps most is known about ankylosing spondylitis. The former England cricket captain Mike Atherton has talked very eloquently about his lifelong battle with this problem during his very successful cricketing career. Among other conditions that are best lumped into this group are tennis elbow and housemaid's knee.

● **Crystal formation within a joint.** The king of this group is by far the best known – gout. Crystals of uric acid develop in the spaces between small joints of the body, typically the big toe, to produce a hot, swollen and exquisitely painful joint.

● **Infection.** I sometimes see what is known as reactive arthritis, where viruses or bacterial organisms find their way into a joint and trigger inflammation, pain and swelling.

One of the problems with arthritis is that it often appears to have a life of its own, flaring up out of the blue. I've no doubt at all that many sufferers are influenced by the weather. One or two of my patients are eerily able to predict the weather for the following 24 hours simply by how their joints feel. My own view is that this phenomenon is linked to barometric pressure, but humidity and temperature also seem to occasionally make symptoms flare up.

Stress is another major trigger, and although it can be almost impossible to remove stress from our lives, if you suffer from arthritis the more you know about looking after your joints the better. Hydrotherapy in the shape of a warm shower or a whirlpool bath can reduce early-morning stiffness and ease aching joints at the end of a long day. Massage can do this too, but you need a qualified practitioner who knows what they are doing and you should always check with your doctor whether the type of arthritis you have can be helped in this way. Relaxation techniques and deep breathing reduce anxiety and in so doing can raise pain thresholds. Many people are not aware that laughter can actually relieve pain – easier said than done, though, if you are in the grip of a bad flare-up of arthritis.

DIET AND ARTHRITIS

I'm often asked whether there is a diet that can help with arthritis. Although the science to support this possibility is sketchy, observation of my patients convinces me that there are ways of eating that can promote a reduction in joint pain and stiffness. It is interesting that the West has a greater incidence of arthritis than, say, Asia, and this has triggered interest in whether diet might play a part here.

In general, if you find that one particular food type seems to make your symptoms worse, avoid it. But whatever food you are eating, you should not be eating so much that you are putting on weight, which is a key enemy when dealing with arthritis. This is especially true of degenerative osteoarthritis as the greater the load a joint has to carry, the more it will complain.

The best basis to start from is a well-balanced diet rich in vegetables, fruits and grains. Then you can look at whether certain food groups can actively reduce inflammation. For this healthy diet we must turn to natural antioxidants. These work by blocking the action of chemicals called free radicals, which are a major factor in causing inflammation in all parts of the body. By blocking free radicals we can help to reduce joint inflammation, and here vitamin E is an important player. This powerful antioxidant can be as effective as conventional treatments in some patients with osteoarthritis. It can do similar things for some people with rheumatoid arthritis, and I find it interesting that some of my patients with this condition have low blood levels of antioxidants compared with the general population. Oily fish such as tuna, mackerel and salmon may also help since these contain omega-3 fatty acids, important in assisting the body's production of prostaglandins, which, in turn, help to control inflammation. Also of frequent benefit in this process are plant seed oils such as evening primrose oil and sunflower seeds.

If you find that it is impractical or unreasonable to have a diet rich in supplements, take a one-a-day multivitamin that contains vitamins A to E as well as folic acid, selenium, magnesium, zinc and copper. In this way you will be giving yourself a good chance of keeping your joints in good condition. Many people with arthritis can also be prone to anaemia, so try to keep your iron levels topped up by eating red meat in moderate amounts, leafy green vegetables and pulses.

As I said earlier, if certain foods seem to make your arthritis worse, avoid them. Time and time again I hear the same suspects mentioned, so you may find it useful to have a list of these:

● **Caffeine.** Many people with arthritis report that tea and coffee seem to increase pain and stiffness.

● **Gluten.** This is found in barley, wheat and oats and is implicated in conditions such as coeliac disease. Some people find that when they cut this out their arthritis dramatically improves, but I would not advocate doing this in the long term if it does not have any clear benefit.

● **Potatoes, tomatoes, peppers and aubergines.** All from the same family, these can trigger arthritis flares.

● **Dairy products.** Milk, butter, cheese and other milk-based foods can also temporarily worsen arthritis.

● **Citrus fruits.** These are among the troublesome foods most often reported to me. Patients say that it is the acidity that aggravates their symptoms and that oranges, lemons and grapefruits have the worst effect. I suspect they are right, but there is no hard science to back this view.

● **Rhubarb.** The oxalic acid in rhubarb inhibits the body's ability to absorb calcium and iron. I've actually seen a bad attack of arthritis occur soon after a meal rich in rhubarb cooked in an aluminium saucepan. You may find rhubarb makes your symptoms worse and so want to avoid it anyway, but if you can eat it, don't use an aluminium pan as the highly acidic juice can dissolve some of the metal, leaving it in the rhubarb.

I'm afraid that trial and error is the order of the day when working out what doesn't suit you, but the pain of giving up some of your favourite foods can be tempered by the knowledge that your arthritic pain should soon start to lessen. If you are a gout sufferer (and you do not need to be a port-swilling lord of the manor to suffer from this), reduce your alcohol intake, increase your general fluid intake and avoid foods rich in purines, which promote the build-up of uric acid in the body. Examples of such foods are offal, anchovies and crab.

MANAGING ARTHRITIS PAIN

If there is one thing that gets arthritis patients down more than anything else, it is the chronic pain. This can often lead to depression, which, in turn, lowers their pain threshold, leading to worse depression in a vicious circle. We each have our own personal ability to tolerate pain, so it's no good listening to what other people say. Just concentrate on what works for you. There are many ways of reducing our pain levels and you need to look at your whole body, as well as your mental state, rather than just focusing on your joints. There is, however, no question that the bedrock of all pain management is medication, and there are many different types on the market to deal with arthritis.

Again, because everybody is different, it can be a process of trial and error before you find the drug that is best for you. Among those most often tried are non-steroidal anti-inflammatory drugs (NSAIDs) such as Ibuprofen, Diclofenac, Naproxen and Indomethacin, but it has been found that simpler drugs such as aspirin and paracetamol can also be very effective here. Discuss with your doctor which drug is right for you as care must be taken that it does not clash with any other medication you are on, or aggravate any pre-existing condition, such as a stomach ulcer.

Compliance with treatment is vital here. I often see patients who request a repeat prescription for their arthritis medication who swear that they take it regularly but get a little confused when I point out that I last gave them their month's supply four months ago. It is important to take painkillers regularly, as this will ensure that you experience less pain than you would by waiting for the pain to arrive and then taking a tablet. Also, if you take the medication only when the pain is especially bad, there can be a problem in linking your drug with pain relief and as a result drug dependence can develop.

Major advances in arthritis drugs have brought alternatives to NSAIDs. These include disease-modifying anti-rheumatic drugs (DMARDs) and Cox inhibitors, both of which are biological response modifiers acting on the proteins that play a major role in rheumatoid arthritis. Steroid tablets can be very effective in controlling flare-ups in rheumatoid arthritis, but these can have marked long-term side effects and so are not normally used for months on end. However, some patients have to stay on them as they are the only drug that controls their symptoms.

Apart from tablets, heat and cold can be effective as well as being very simple to use. A cold pack may not be a good idea if you have heart or circulation problems, so check with your doctor first. But if you are able to use one, ice can be very effective in relieving the pain and swelling of inflamed joints caused by rheumatoid arthritis. The cold constricts blood vessels beneath the skin and so prevents fluids leaking into surrounding tissues. Take frozen peas, or ice cubes in a freezer bag, out of the freezer and wrap them in a clean tea towel. Place this ice pack on the affected joint for 10–15 minutes, but keep checking to make sure that the skin does not go red or blotchy as this can be a sign that it is too cold. This can be repeated every three hours or so, and if you want to achieve a deeper cold penetration, add moisture. To do this wet a towel with warm water before wrapping up the ice pack and then apply it. This can also reduce the risk of over-cooling or freezing the tissues.

If you want to try a heat pack, again check with your doctor that this is a suitable option for you. I find the microwaveable oat bags available from chemist's and health shops extremely useful here. They are quick to prepare, easy to apply, reusable and very effective. Twenty minutes' application is normally long enough to get results, after which you can leave the pack off for two or three hours before reuse. Here again pain relief can be increased if moisture is added; just place the heat pack in a plastic bag and then wrap it in a damp towel before use.

We take our natural movements and flexibility for granted, so it can be a shock if we start to stiffen or our joints begin to ache when we are doing simple tasks. If you begin to suffer from arthritis it is sensible to give yourself regular breaks when working on activities that might overstress joints, and doing this should also lessen the risk of accidents. Never ignore pain or signs of inflammation, as this means your body is telling you that you may need to either temporarily slow down or alter the way you are working. Pace yourself and rest if you are able to. Simple tips such as lifting correctly, always using both hands to lift heavy objects and leaning into a heavy door rather than opening it with your hands are common sense but often forgotten.

Stay as active as possible. Your joints are meant to be used and the best forms of exercise here are walking, swimming and stretching such as is found in yoga or t'ai chi, since all these place only gentle pressure on muscles and the surrounding joints. Running or treadmill work is probably best avoided because of the strain they put on joints. For both your physical and mental well-being it is best to exercise little and often. Avoid activities that use one position for a long time whenever possible, and take frequent breaks or stretch at regular intervals to reduce the likelihood of stiffness developing.

OSTEOPOROSIS

Although it is a well-known fact that 27.6% of statistics are made up, I occasionally come across one that really makes me sit up and think. One such figure is that every three minutes in the UK someone has a fractured bone as a result of osteoporosis. So, depending on your reading speed, by the time you have read this chapter some two to four people will be suffering from a fracture that was not there when you started it. About one in twelve men (and one in three women) in this country will develop this problem during their lifetime and an estimated three million people suffer from it, most of them having no idea there is anything wrong. With the financial state of the NHS rarely out of the headlines, the little matter of osteoporosis costing over £1.5 billion each year is not exactly small change either.

So much for the size of the problem, but what exactly is osteoporosis? The literal meaning, porous bones, gives a clue. Our bones are made up of a strong outer shell and a honeycomb-like centre in which blood vessels and bone marrow lie. When these tiny holes inside the bone become bigger, it becomes more fragile and so more likely to break. For most people of either sex loss of what is called bone density, a natural part of ageing, does not begin until after about 35.

Men are not as resistant to this problem, also known as bone thinning, as was once thought, but the types of fractures that become more likely with age tend to happen less in a man because of his larger skeletal mass. Other factors include shorter male life expectancy (the longer you live, the thinner the bones and the greater the risk of fractures), slower progress of bone destruction and the absence of the rapid bone thinning that often occurs in women as a result of the menopause. The plain truth, though, is that the chances of male osteoporosis developing do increase with age, with the lifetime risk of low-trauma hip, back or wrist fracture being as high as 13% in a 50-year-old man and 25% by the time he reaches 60. It has been estimated that around 30% of hip fractures worldwide are in men, with their mortality rate in the first post-fracture month being as high as 12%, compared with 5% in women. And if we look at X-rays of men's backs, the prevalence of radiographic vertebral deformities linked to osteoporosis – once considered uncommon – is found to be higher in men under 65 than in women under that age.

CAUSES OF MALE OSTEOPOROSIS

The main causes of osteoporosis in men are:

● Idiopathic osteoporosis, which means that there is no obvious detectable or identifiable cause. About a third of cases fall into in this category and in these patients a strong family history of the condition is not uncommon.
● Ageing, which causes loss of bone density.
● Alcohol. There is a definite link between heavy drinking and bone thinning, although the exact reason why one triggers the other remains unclear. A number of factors come into play here, including an increased risk of trauma, dietary deficiencies and a reduction in the activity of osteoblastic cells, which are crucial for maintaining bone density.
● Long-term use of steroid tablets (often for conditions such as asthma or inflammatory bowel disease) increases

the risk. Steroids reduce levels of the male hormone testosterone in the body as well as affecting osteoblastic cells.

- Hormonal problems linked to hypogonadism. Here male hormones do not strengthen the bones as they should, so their density declines.
- Kidney stones. Several reports have linked formation of calcium kidney stones to reduced bone density in men.

Because bone thinning can't be felt or seen, most people with osteoporosis are not aware of any problem until they suffer a fracture, and so it is truly one of the 'silent' diseases. Although X-rays readily show up broken bones, osteoporosis only becomes apparent when at least 30% of the bone density has been lost. This means accurate assessment is needed, and here the best solution is a bone density scan called a Dual Energy X-ray Absorptiometry (DXA) scan. This scan is recommended for people who are at high risk of osteoporosis, but its availability varies widely across the country and your GP will need to assess your medical history before considering a referral. Results of the scan show how your bone density compares with the average for your age and sex, and therefore whether bone thinning is present.

To lessen your chances of getting to that stage, you can take preventive measures. The first is to begin to strengthen your skeleton with a bone-friendly diet, rich in calcium, based on sources such as cheese, milk and yoghurt. Fortunately, low-fat varieties of these contain just as much calcium as the fuller-fat ones. Don't forget that bread, green leafy vegetables, oily fish and tofu are also rich in calcium. Take care not to eat too much salt or drink lots of caffeine-containing drinks as these can reduce calcium absorption.

Vitamin D is needed to help calcium uptake in the body. Sunshine is the best source of this – enjoying 20 minutes of sunlight daily during summer can enable the body to store enough vitamin D to last the rest of the year. (If for any reason diet is a problem, an acceptable alternative is calcium supplements.) The Department of Health recommends a daily adult calcium intake of 700 milligrams, but the National Osteoporosis Society suggest a higher intake may be slightly more beneficial.

It is not only diet that is useful here, for exercise also plays a key role in keeping bones strong and healthy. This can range from brisk walking to swimming or cycling, but whatever the preferred activity it is important that it is performed for at least 20 minutes three or four times a week. The benefit of exercise is shown by the fact that tennis players have a 30% higher bone density in their serving arm compared with their non-serving one, and joggers have higher than average bone density in their spines. Even jumping on the spot 50–60 times a day can increase bone density.

TREATMENT FOR OSTEOPOROSIS

Sadly for us all, once bone density has decreased it can't be replaced completely and treatment is therefore always aimed at helping to prevent further bone loss. Various treatments are available, including parathyroid hormone replacement therapy, calcium and vitamin D supplements (guidelines suggest 1,200 milligrams of calcium and 500 IU of vitamin D daily for people over 50) and testosterone treatment, although the benefit of this in ageing men needs to be set against its theoretically adverse effect on the prostate gland.

Compared with those for women, there have been few trials of therapies specifically for osteoporotic men, but drugs such as Alendronate and Risedronate – non-hormonal treatments which work by switching off the cells that break down bone – appear to significantly increase bone density.

There are few conditions to which the tenet 'prevention is better than cure' applies more accurately than osteoporosis. Fortunately, for most people the best medicine is a healthy lifestyle with plenty of sunshine, exercise and a sensible diet.

KEY POINTS

- Arthritis causes considerable problems in large numbers of men.
- The commonest type is osteoarthritis.
- There are many ways to treat it, including diet, drugs and natural treatments.
- Many specialists now recommend glucosamine as an alternative to conventional anti-inflammatory drugs.
- Osteoporosis is more common in men than first realised.
- It is a 'silent' illness, often first noticed when a bone breaks.
- Prevention of osteoporosis is possible in the majority of men by stopping smoking, eating an appropriate diet, exercising regularly, cutting down on alcohol and supplementing inadequate levels of calcium and vitamin D.

9

DEMENTIA

'Honey, I forgot to duck ...'
– **President Reagan** *to his wife after being shot*

Many men over 50 are concerned about becoming demented in later life, but when I quiz them closely I find there is often a great deal of misunderstanding and inappropriate anxiety about the issue. In a nutshell, dementia is an excessive steady decline in all areas of mental ability and is therefore an illness of the brain. In dementia the brain cells die faster than they would as part of the normal ageing process and this loss of excess amounts of brain cells means that the brain does not work as it should. Over time a person with dementia loses the ability to do simple things, but it is a myth that the condition is a natural part of ageing. It is not, and symptoms suggestive of dementia need thorough investigation regardless of a person's age.

It is encouraging to know that most old people will never get any form of dementia. It affects about 5% of people over the age of 65, rising to some 20% of those over 80. It is not infectious and it is not caused by stress or anxiety or too little or too much mental activity. According to an estimate made by the Alzheimer's Society, some 750,000 people in the UK suffer from dementia and this number is expected to gradually increase over the next two decades as a consequence of the population living longer.

TYPES OF DEMENTIA

Dementia is a multi-factorial illness, which means that there are a number of causes. However, most cases fall into one of four main types: Alzheimer's disease, vascular dementia, Lewy body dementia and alcohol-related dementia. Let's consider these individually:

● **Alzheimer's disease.** Perhaps the best known and commonest type of dementia, this is categorised as either early-onset or late-onset, meaning, respectively, the illness begins before the age of 65 and after 65. In the UK about 70% of people of this age and over who have dementia have Alzheimer's disease and, although there is no single gene responsible for it, there is evidence in many cases of a genetic link. In early-onset Alzheimer's there can be problems with chromosome numbers 14 and 21 and about half of the children of someone with one of these particular abnormalities inherit it and so may go on to develop Alzheimer's. However, this defect does not skip a generation, so if you don't inherit it you can't pass it on to your children. If you are very unfortunate and have three or more close relatives who developed the disease between the ages of 35 and 60, you should be referred by your GP to a specialist for genetic testing of familial Alzheimer's.

In late-onset Alzheimer's there is a weaker genetic link than in early-onset Alzheimer's, but the first affects more people. Although the science is dull, it is worth understanding a little of it. The genes involved are Apo E3 and Apo E4.

Some 2% of the population inherit two Apo E4 genes from their parents, and this makes them 16 times more likely to develop Alzheimer's. Twenty-five per cent of the population inherit one Apo E4 gene, which increases their risk of developing Alzheimer's by a factor of four. Sixty per cent of the population inherit two Apo E3 genes, but this only puts them at an average risk of developing Alzheimer's and about half of those with two such genes have developed the disease by their late eighties.

No significant link has yet been proven between the environment and dementia. There is circumstantial evidence of a link between Alzheimer's disease and both aluminium and mercury, but the link is not proven in either case. Although aluminium has been shown to be associated with some of the characteristic findings in the brains of Alzheimer's patients, there is still no clear evidence that it has actually caused the illness. Mercury has been used in dental fillings and is a substance poisonous to the body, but once again there is no proven link with Alzheimer's.

Not only does Alzheimer's destroy brain cells, but in doing so it disrupts the chemical neuro-transmitters that transport information in the brain. This is why memory and other mental abilities become affected, and the brain damage that occurs is caused by two main problems. The first is the threads of proteins, known as tangles, that develop within cells in the brain; the second is the so-called plaques that occur between brain cells.

Even while President Ronald Reagan was in office at the White House, his slow delivery and sometimes odd choice of words had many people questioning whether there was more to his mental condition than the normal effects of ageing. As his verbal dexterity and memory continued to wane he publicly and bravely announced he was suffering from Alzheimer's before retiring from office and withdrawing from the public eye. The former Prime Minister Harold Wilson – one of the most astute political beasts of any colour in the past century – also succumbed to this disease. He had a family history of Alzheimer's and was aware of its early symptoms, so it must have been particularly cruel when he first became aware of its strengthening grip on him. Shortly before he died he gave an interview to a journalist on *The Times*, during which he admitted that he could not remember any details of his last government and that by the time he had read to the bottom of a page he had forgotten the start of it.

● **Vascular dementias, including multi-infarct dementia.** This type of dementia is the commonest type after Alzheimer's disease and accounts for up to 20% of all other cases of dementia. It is caused by damage to the blood vessels that lead to the brain and supply it with oxygen. If there is poor circulation of blood to the brain, the oxygen supply is cut off and brain cells die. In multi-infarct dementia a lot of mini-strokes can occur which cut off the blood supply to part of the brain. Strokes are a well-recognised cause of vascular dementia and they are also associated with weakness or paralysis on one side of the body, along with a loss of balance and disturbed vision or speech. Multi-infarct dementia can be progressive, exhibiting what seem to be a series of dizzy spells which, in fact, develop into growing confusion and dementia of this type over a period of months or years.

● **Lewy body dementia.** This accounts for about 15% of cases other than Alzheimer's and is named after the tiny protein structures that develop inside nerve cells in the brains of affected people. It is these that destroy the brain tissue and so affect concentration, language and memory. People with this type of dementia may be more prone to seeing things (visual hallucinations) as well as having spells of abnormal behaviour and unsteadiness. In my experience people with this type of dementia seem particularly prone to the side effects of drugs used to treat dementia in general.

● **Alcohol-related dementia.** This is the least common type of dementia, but it is an inescapable fact that excess alcohol taken over a long time can cause significant brain damage. The progression of this dementia is directly linked to both quantity and duration of alcohol abuse. Stopping drinking completely is the only treatment here.

SYMPTOMS OF DEMENTIA

Dementia is a progressive illness, which means that it usually worsens over time, but the early symptoms tend to include memory loss and forgetting simple but important facts such as even a close relative's name or birthday or other significant dates. There is often confusion about where that person is in time or space and there may be difficulty in recalling certain words, although this alone is not a sign of dementia as we are all forgetful from time to time. As the disease progresses, the sufferer may become listless and lose interest in activities which they previously considered important. There is often a degree of emotional disturbance, with mood swings and sometimes depression. In the later stages people can lose the ability to look after themselves completely and so need help

129

with washing, dressing and eating. Conversation may become utterly repetitive, with the patient asking the same question over and over again. The personality may disintegrate and although the person may be completely unaware of their plight (which is often a blessing), this aspect of dementia can be particularly distressing for their carers.

It is important to realise that it is quite normal to forget something but still remember details associated with it and that this is not a dementing process. For most people, as they age, forgetfulness is simply a damn nuisance, but this alone is not dementia. One simple way of confirming this is to think of your next-door neighbour. You may forget their name on occasion but you will still know that they are your neighbour. By contrast, people with dementia not only forget the person's name but are completely unaware of the fact that they are their neighbour and may even be unaware that they have ever seen them before. Generally, dementia usually takes six to nine months to become apparent and it is often a partner or close relative who first notices changes in behaviour. However, accurate diagnosis is vital here and I do not diagnose dementia without referring the patient to a specialist such as a psycho-geriatrician.

There can be other possible causes of symptoms similar to dementia, including depression and thyroid problems. In such cases diagnostic tests include verbal tests and brief mental state tests which are repeated after several months to see if there is any change in mental ability, as well as brain scanning to check if other problems, such as brain tumours, are present or if parts of the brain are shrinking. Newer and more costly tests are now assisting in the diagnosis of Alzheimer's and these include positron emission tomography (PET), which assesses the metabolism of the brain, and single photon emission computerised tomography (SPECT), which it is hoped will help doctors identify treatable and non-treatable causes of dementia. An electro-encephalogram (EEG) can be used to measure the electrical activity in the brain, since abnormally slow activity can indicate Alzheimer's. However, because this may also show normal electrical brain activity, it is not in itself diagnostic but simply one of a series of tests.

None of these tests is painful, but they can be upsetting for both the patient and relatives, especially if the patient has insight into what the diagnosis might be. It may also be a considerable time before a diagnosis is made, and this, in turn, is often stressful.

Depression, very common in the elderly, often masquerades as a dementing process and this condition, known as pseudo-dementia, can fool even the most authoritative of specialists.

CAN DEMENTIA BE PREVENTED?

Sadly, there is little that can be done to prevent any geneti-cally linked dementia from developing with time, but one area where lifestyle changes can be beneficial is with the vascular dementias. Anything that can be done to reduce vascular disease and strokes linked with this type of dementia is to be encouraged. Therefore, if you smoke you should stop, if you do not take regular exercise you should start to do so and you should make sure that your blood pressure is satisfactory and your cholesterol level normal. Encouragingly for me, a modest alcohol intake is probably beneficial here. Research in Australia found that army recruits who were moderate consumers of alcohol were less likely to develop

Alzheimer's 40 or 50 years later than either their heavy-drinking or their teetotal counterparts. Subsequent European research has backed up these findings, so a glass or two of red wine a day seems to be no bad thing here.

I'm often asked whether staying mentally active can help prevent or delay dementia. The evidence is not clear-cut, but I've no doubt that if you have a generally good intellect and continue to use this in old age, you are less likely to develop early Alzheimer's disease. It is not enough just to read, though – you need to be using your creative brain by writing, doing crosswords or similar puzzles or learning new skills such as computing. I have a handful of professional patients in their seventies and eighties who, I'm convinced, remain as mentally alert as they do precisely because they continue to exercise their brain as they would their body. As one of them said to me recently, 'Far better to wear out than rust out.'

Unfortunately, there is no cure for Alzheimer's, since once brain cells have been destroyed they cannot be replaced, so damage is permanent. Any treatment that is given tends only to delay the onset of symptoms and the exact form this takes depends on the type of dementia diagnosed. Treatment is now part of a team approach and this team usually includes, in addition to the family doctor, consultant psycho-geriatricians, occupational, language and speech therapists and specialist nurses. The principal aim of treatment is to sustain as much physical and mental ability for as long as possible. We must remember here that in many people with dementia the symptoms may well remain minor for a number of years. When these occur the person should not be treated like a child or as slow-witted. Patronising those with mild dementia can be extremely insulting to them and may even worsen any symptoms of anxiety and depression they are already feeling following diagnosis. Speech and language therapists are used to help sufferers make better use of their existing brain cells, occupational therapists can be very effective in helping them to cope better at home with their everyday activities and art or music therapy may also prove beneficial. The burden placed on carers or relatives is often so heavy that they themselves may experience depression. This is where respite care is so useful, allowing dementia patients to attend a day centre or day hospital for breaks which help carers and relatives lead as normal a life as possible.

MEDICATION

The majority of medications employed to treat dementia are those used for Alzheimer's disease. Other medications aim to treat associated symptoms of dementia, such as insomnia, anxiety, depression and hallucinations, and most are of the antidepressant or anxiolytic (anti-anxiety) type. Aspirin is often used to keep the risk of strokes to a minimum and by this means to try to delay progression of a vascular dementia.

Drugs used for Alzheimer's are intended not only to treat some of the symptoms but also to slow the progression of the disease, and these are best given early in the illness. These are specialist treatments and should be monitored by a consultant as they can have significant side effects, including nausea and loss of appetite, fatigue and diarrhoea. Two such drugs that I commonly deal with are Aricept (donepezil hydrochloride) and Exelon (Rivastigmine), which act directly on the brains of Alzheimer's sufferers. One of the main problems here is that Alzheimer's patients have depleted levels of acetylcholine – vital in maintaining effective nerve cell memory and communication. These two drugs aim to maintain levels of this chemical by blocking the production of a particular enzyme that acts to remove it. By helping the brain to make better use of its healthy brain cells to do this, they can stabilise or reduce symptoms of Alzheimer's in the early stages for some months. But, and this is a big but, the cost of these drugs is a massive issue for health authorities in the UK, and limited budgets often restrict the ability of specialists to prescribe them. This is currently a hot potato in clinical medicine and we can only watch this space to see how it develops. I get very frustrated when deserving patients have had to resort to funding their own treatment out of desperation.

If you believe you have symptoms suggestive of dementia, do not be too embarrassed or worried to discuss this with your doctor, as very often such fears are misplaced. At the same time, it is far better to know about any problems sooner rather than later, in order to be able to plan ahead and maintain the best quality of life possible.

KEY POINTS

- Dementia is an excessive steady decline in all mental activity, its effects intensifying with age.
- Dementia affects about 5% of people over 65 and about 20% of those over 80.
- The commonest type of dementia is Alzheimer's disease, which accounts for over two-thirds of all cases.
- Alzheimer's which occurs before the age of 65 is described as early-onset; when it occurs after this age it is described as late-onset.

● **Treatment of dementia is possible in certain cases, but only in early dementia and then as a palliative rather than a cure.**

10
THE MALE MENOPAUSE

'The only way to keep your health is to eat what you don't want, drink what you don't like, and do what you'd rather not.'
– **Mark Twain**

If there is one male condition that tends to split doctors into separate camps it is the so-called male menopause, formally referred to as the andropause. Here I will put my hand up straight away and say that I don't believe that the male menopause exists in men as a distinct clinical entity in the same way that the female menopause does. I don't deny, however, that many men do experience some degree of mid-life crisis, which is what most people mean when they talk about the male menopause. There are some specialists who claim that the two are different and that the male menopause is purely down to a diminishing supply of sex hormones. I believe, though, that the majority of the symptoms that can develop in a male mid-life crisis are psychological, but that in some men the process can be accelerated by rapidly falling levels of the testosterone hormone.

Between the late thirties and about 55 is the age of most of the men I see who conform to stereotype by either chucking their wife for a younger model or leave their job to travel the world. Hard statistics are almost impossible to come by here, but some specialists who believe in the existence of the male menopause say that perhaps 25% of 50-year-olds suffer from it to some degree. For the men who visit me, work is their main source of personal identity. Many have given little thought to the major events of life such as ageing, retirement and children leaving home and marrying. If you throw into the mix divorce and changes in sexual function, you have a set of circumstances in which a man can start to experience typical symptoms.

The most frequently reported problems are:

- Loss of sex drive, or impotence
- Marked fatigue
- Irritability and outbursts of anger
- Feelings of lethargy, sadness or depression
- Occasional bursts of greater activity than normal in an attempt to avoiding feeling old

There may also be more vague symptoms such as night sweats, general joint and muscle stiffness, eczema, weight gain and hair loss. Many of these symptoms are normal consequences of ageing, but the fact is that by middle age most men are likely to have achieved their realistic goals in life and yet be feeling unclear about where they are going in the future. In addition, children leaving the parental home can add to anxiety and insecurity. Poor sleep is a factor which is often associated with a male mid-life crisis but which tends to be forgotten here. Men in their late forties tend to sleep far more lightly than when they were younger, with fewer episodes of the REM sleep in which our bodies recharge their batteries the fastest. By a linked hormonal process, inadequate sleep may also contribute to the weight gain that so many middle-aged men experience.

Bearing in mind the often pronounced psychological aspect of a male mid-life crisis, what, on the other hand, is the argument for a hormonal imbalance causing the problem? Well, some experts attribute the symptoms to a decrease in testosterone, the male hormone responsible for sexual characteristics and sex drive. Although the level of testosterone in the body starts to gradually lessen from our late twenties and continues to fall thereafter, this is a very different pattern from the loss of oestrogen in women. Oestrogen drops suddenly, usually in the mid to late forties, and this triggers the female menopause. This abrupt and marked change does not happen with testosterone in men and is a real spanner in the works for those who try to explain the mid-life crisis in purely hormonal terms.

However, playing devil's advocate, I suggest that a case can be made for the central role of hormones. It goes something like this: as men get older their blood contains more of the substance called sex hormone binding globulin (SHBG) and this appears to increase in middle-aged men. As it does so it binds to testosterone, with the result that this cannot be used by the body. So, as men get older, it is not so much that they have a dramatically low level of testosterone in the blood but rather that the amount available for use has fallen significantly.

In addition, the body's cells, including those that make up so-called male tissues, which are influenced by testosterone, may develop thicker walls with age, so that they are less able to absorb testosterone. This, in theory at least, could explain why the testosterone level in an andropausal man is often found to be normal when effectively it is not.

If, like me, you believe that the vast majority of men who experience a mid-life crisis have primarily a psychological problem, bear in mind that there are steps that can be taken to head off the problem, as well as ways of getting through it when it does strike. The first thing to do is take the hard step and accept that, although 40 may be the old age of youth, you should think of 50 as being the youth of old age. Many men believe that as they get older their horizons narrow and they have to do less and less. I believe the reverse is true. With current medical knowledge as it is, even at the age of 60 you may only be two-thirds of the way through your life and that leaves a huge amount of time to broaden your interests, learn new skills or travel widely. Think of ageing as an opportunity to constantly re-evaluate your life and, if it feels necessary, change direction or branch out into new areas.

At this time it is also important to resist the temptation to fall back on alcohol or nicotine to ease stress, as these will only make the problem worse in the long term. I've discussed exercise many times in this book but again and again I see it proved to be one of the most effective ways of relaxing the body as well as promoting a positive mood and reducing mild depression. You might also look at other alternative therapies, such as massage, yoga or acupuncture, as a way of reducing stress and aiding relaxation.

Men are notoriously reluctant to talk about their problems and they often find this all the harder the better they know someone. Talking to a complete stranger can help here, so if you request it, your GP may be able to refer you to a counsellor so that you can discuss problems such as impotence, relationship difficulties or other issues that can trouble a man's middle years.

Make sure you are eating well and having regular, relaxed meals through the day rather than eating on the hoof or missing meals altogether. Try to keep food as pure as possible by avoiding too many refined sugars and saturated fats (fats which are solid at room temperature, such as butter and lard). It is often helpful at times of stress to supplement your diet with vitamins such as vitamin B complex.

Don't hang on to the fact that when you were young you may have been able to swing from the chandelier all night for nights on end and still work a 16-hour day before winning the World Cup for England in your lunch break. Sex changes as we age but don't fight this. Explore it, use it as a way of finding real intimacy with your partner, as this often provides far more satisfying sex than you have previously had. Go for quality rather than quantity.

Remember perspective in your life. This theme crops up repeatedly when I'm discussing patients' stress levels with them, and it is surely no coincidence that Britons work the longest hours in Europe yet report the least job satisfaction. Take a long, hard look at what is truly necessary in your life and whenever possible cut down on your working hours and spend more time with your family and friends. You may be able to do this by developing better time-management skills, not taking on work you strictly do not have to do and learning to delegate appropriately. Try giving the same amount of time and effort to family and friends as you do to your work. Many men are terrifically proud of their bursting appointment diaries but would not think of putting the same amount of effort into nurturing the relationships that they know somewhere are the most important thing in their life.

TESTOSTERONE REPLACEMENT THERAPY

Returning to the role that hormones might play, if the whole issue of the male menopause causes friction between doctors, then the use of testosterone positively sets it alight. Basically this involves giving supplementary testosterone, by means of injections, patches, tablets or creams, to men suffering from symptoms that suggest the andropause. I've sometimes noted advocates of testosterone replacement therapy (TRT) refer to it as 'the testosterone feelgood factor'. According to its advocates, many men who have received TRT report significant improvements in their well-being, including a stronger sex drive, increased energy, less irritability and a general ability to cope far better with life than previously. But if this is such a wonder drug, why is it not being used on every grumpy middle-aged man?

Well, we come back to the question of whether or not the male menopause actually exists as a clinical condition. If, as I believe, it does not occur in the majority of men, TRT may simply be an attempt to provide an instant fix for a problem that is actually normal but with which men are experiencing difficulty. Simply shoving hormones into a man while ignoring fundamental psychological issues is going about it the wrong way, since these problems remain unaddressed and therefore untreated.

Call me a cynic if you will, but I've noticed that the greatest advocates of TRT in my profession are often doctors in private practice – the treatment is usually provided by private clinics rather than on the NHS – and I wonder whether they would be shouting quite as loudly if they were not receiving the odd penny or two from dispensing it.

There is also a significant issue concerning testosterone and prostate cancer, although there is little good evidence that testosterone actually initiates this form of cancer. Nevertheless, there is a body of work that suggests that testosterone can promote it once it is there; in other words, it can be petrol on the fire. So any man who has been given TRT should be having regular checks of his prostate, at least every six months. At present there is also little good evidence of the long-term safety and efficacy of TRT. While this argument could be applied to a number of drugs currently on the market, it does not mean that testosterone should not be used with considerable care.

I fully accept that complementary practitioners are often more willing to accept the notion of the andropause than hard-nosed conventional medics like myself and, provided the treatment given to a patient is safe, I've no problem with it at all. Examples of this for men include evening primrose oil, which helps to regulate body processes in general, and borage, which is said to support the adrenal glands and so reduce strain on the hormonal system.

No matter who is right in the male menopause debate, ultimately a man going through a mid-life crisis must himself answer a number of questions and these all boil down to his ability to manage change of one kind or another. By the time they reach their sixties, most men have realised and accepted where they are going in life, but the ones who really do well are those who realise that fresh perspectives and challenges are always out there and should always be sought. Forget life beginning at forty. It can begin at any age you choose and sitting in misery believing that life has somehow passed you by is most definitely bad for your health.

KEY POINTS

- It is hotly debated whether the male menopause exists.
- For many, if not most, men, the late forties and early fifties are a time of major reappraisal of their life.

- **The majority of middle-aged men experience psychological stress, usually linked to important changes such as redundancy, problems in their relationship with their partner or younger colleagues or their children leaving home.**
- **A very small number may have symptoms attributable to testosterone deficiency.**

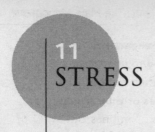

11
STRESS

'When Martina Navratilova is tense, it helps her relax.'
– **Dan Maskell**, *commentating at Wimbledon*

If there is one word I hear more than any other in my surgery it's 'stress'. Up to a half of all my consultations concern stress-related problems, and stress is used as a reason for so much that is wrong in the world that it has become an almost meaningless cliché. But ask yourself this: if you were transported back 100 years, would you know what stress was? To be sure, there was probably more basic hardship and certainly more suffering due to illness but stress as a concept was almost unknown apart from vague references to 'nervous prostration' or 'a fit of the vapours'. The irony is that people then had exactly the same reaction to stress as we do today – they could hardly fail to do otherwise since our body design has not changed in that time.

When faced with a situation we perceive as stressful – and we must always remember that this perception varies massively between individuals – our bodies prepare to combat it by releasing hormones. These powerful chemicals in the form of adrenalin and noradrenalin increase our heart rate, raise our blood pressure and dilate our eyes in order that we can meet the challenge – the so-called 'fight or flight' reaction. In the days when we hunted for food we could put this to good use by, say, killing dangerous animals more efficiently or running faster when we had to escape a tricky situation. Now we are more likely to be sitting fuming in a traffic jam, releasing the same hormones but without being able to use them. The result? Good old-fashioned 'stress' but with a 'modern' feel to it.

Of all the different definitions of stress, the best ones contain the word 'change'. Anything that our bodies perceive as being unusual or a break with routine may trigger a stress reaction. The irony is that we cannot live without stress – it gets us out of bed in the mornings and keeps us functioning through the day. A life without stress would be terminally dull, but if we are constantly exposed to what we believe is too much change we may experience the physical and mental symptoms we all know – headaches, muscle tension, diarrhoea, shallow breathing and so on.

Short burst of stress are not dangerous. Adrenalin and other stress-linked hormones are released into the body to allow us to deal with the immediate problem or get away as fast as we can. Longer-term or chronic stress, however, is a different problem. Although it isn't a killer in itself, it is probably a risk factor for developing heart problems in later life, and if it is allowed to continue unchecked it undoubtedly worsens other health problems, such as insomnia, irritable bowel syndrome, psoriasis and migraines. The exact reasons for this prolonged stress remain unclear but the pace of life nowadays means that many people find it increasingly difficult to 'switch off' from the pressures and so feel unwell as a result.

What are the telltale signs of stress? There are too many to list here, but the ones I see most often are:

- Not being able to sleep properly and lying awake worrying about everything
- Poor concentration and increased irritability
- Drinking more caffeine and/or alcohol than usual, and/or smoking more
- Inability to make decisions, which increases frustration
- Palpitations of the heart, a 'lump' in the throat or stomach, a dry mouth and slight tremor of the hands
- A constant feeling that something needs to be done and that you cannot simply sit and relax by doing nothing

DEALING WITH STRESS

So what can you do to reduce the stress in your life? Here are some of the most effective ways to lessen its effects:

● **Keep a stress diary.** Keep a diary, for at least a fortnight, of events, times, places and people that seem to make you more stressed. You may well be surprised to find that a pattern soon emerges and this may be linked to time pressure, personality clashes, inappropriate demands being made on you or simply trying to do too many things at once. Even just seeing your problems in black and white can make you feel more in control of your life. Once you have worked out the sources of stress or conflict, talk through your diary with your partner or a close friend. Ask for impartial advice on how to ease the problems you have discovered. Another person's perspective will often shed a lot of light on where you are going wrong.

● **Learn how to relax.** Where practical, before you enter known stressful situations of the kinds you have identified, use the following relaxation techniques. Practise deep breathing by inhaling slowly through your nose while counting to five, holding your breath for five seconds and then exhaling slowly through slightly parted lips. Repeat this ten times when feeling stressed, focusing completely on your breathing.

Stretch the muscles of your neck and shoulders by keeping your shoulders level and trying to touch each shoulder with your ear. Look right up at the ceiling, down at the floor and then rotate each shoulder in a wide circle. Repeat this five times. Open and close your jaw widely after each time since stress often causes tension in this area.

● **Exercise regularly.** You don't have to be a gym freak to get the stress-busting benefits of exercise. Even 20 minutes of brisk walking three times a week will help to reduce stress as well as promoting restful sleep.

● **Plan 'firebreaks' in your day.** Allow time for the unexpected (which, of course, will happen). Get up 15 minutes earlier than you think you need to and prepare for the day without rushing. Better still, get everything ready the night before. Try to have 20 minutes in the morning and again in the afternoon that is exclusively 'your' time in which you can do whatever you want even if it is simply sitting doing nothing. When things get busy, look forward to these times you have earmarked for yourself. If on occasion it really is impossible to take advantage of them, always 'catch up' later.

● **Take time out.** If you absolutely can't take a longer break, you should at least 'shut down' for five minutes every hour or two and focus your mind on your perfect situation. This could be a dream holiday or your ideal partner or simply thinking about doing nothing at all. You will be surprised at how effectively this can lower stress levels.

● **Don't use alcohol and smoking as crutches.** In the long term these simply make stress worse. Drinking more to 'calm your nerves' is a slippery slope. Smoking more simply intensifies all the health problems associated with the habit (which are discussed in detail in the following chapter).

SOURCES OF STRESS

Each of us reacts differently to the complex set of factors that produce stress. It is only by recognising where your individual stresses are coming from and then acting on these problems that you can relieve stress and improve your emotional and physical well-being. However, there are certain stressful situations that men tend to find themselves in, so let's look at these as templates for action. In no particular order, here are the five most common sources of stress at work, followed by two frequent problems connected with stress generated outside the workplace:

● **Boss stress.** If your boss is impossible to get on with, you have a choice. If there are specific issues that are causing problems, raise these with him or her and suggest possible solutions. If your boss will not listen you may have to accept that your work will suffer as a result but that this is not your fault. It is vital to focus on *functions*, not personalities. Remember that resigning need not be a failure and can actually show strength on your part. Always bear in mind the golden rule: if the situation cannot change, change your reaction to it.

● **Colleague stress.** The key to dealing with people who are aggressive or devious at work is to be assertive without becoming aggressive yourself. Remember:

- Always try to be straight with people – they may not like what you say but they will always know where they stand with you.
- Have a relaxed, open body stance rather than a defensive one such as arms crossed or pointing your finger in someone's face.
- Even if you disagree radically with the other person, always listen to them. You will have more chance of convincing someone if they feel you have listened to them rather than closed your ears or blustered.
- State your case consistently, repeating it if necessary. Never allow yourself to be distracted by the other person's arguments – they may know they are wrong and be trying to deflect you from your persuasive argument.
- Silence can be extremely effective. Don't fall into the trap of assuming you have to answer every argument. A thoughtful silence followed by the one word 'No' can be extremely effective.

● **'Fraud' stress.** We all occasionally think we are no good at what we do and worry that somehow we are going to be 'found out' and sacked on the spot. Bearing in mind that most of the other people you work with are thinking the same thing about themselves, the trick here is to play to your strengths. First, you will need to recognise these. Write down all the strengths you think you have. Do not be too critical or modest. Then ask a few good friends to do the same about you, and compare the lists. You may not believe you have particular skills, but if a number of people say you do, they will not all be mistaken or lying to flatter you. You may even find you are neglecting talents you have and that you can use these to improve your work prospects.

● **Presentation stress.** The key to this common problem is the three Ps – Panic, Prepare, Present. First, remember that anxiety is normal. Everyone feels anxious about speaking in public even if they do not show it. This nervousness usually increases the nearer you get to the big day, so accept this will happen and there is little you can do about it. Secondly, prepare. Most people's anxiety is due to a fear of the unknown. Preparing well in advance kills this fear – read your speech until you know it backwards and can imagine yourself giving it with confidence. Don't ignore any weak areas you feel you may have, such as a topic you think you may get caught out on. Review thoroughly everything you need to know, not just your strong areas. Finally, present. Rather than thinking about everyone watching you, focus on one person in the room and aim to speak to them alone without making it too obvious that this is what you are doing. It is much less stressful to feel you are speaking one to one than to a room full of people.

● **Techno stress.** When it comes to coping with the changing demands of computers and software, for most of us it is a matter of knowing how to ask for help. I'm assuming that you have spent a little time with a user manual but still have questions, although it is surprising how many people find even this stressful and give up on it. Don't assume that others are necessarily more adept at handling technology than you are – they will have simply discovered, or been told, which keys to press to carry out particular tasks. Flattery often plays a big part here, as you may need to pander to egos to get the assistance you need. Go to a colleague you get on with and say something like, 'What tricks do you use to get around your computer like you do?' or, 'Could you show me some tips to help me with this project?' Naturally, this is more likely to work within a team rather than in a situation where individuals are simply sharing the same workspace. Even then, it never does any harm to be honest and ask in a friendly way for advice.

● **Time stress.** When many people say, 'I haven't got the time', what they often mean is, 'I haven't got the time given the way I choose to spend it.' Take last week's TV guide and circle any programme you watched. Now try to remember every one. Still think you use your time properly? Aim to keep 'work pollution' of your leisure time to a minimum by targeting two days each week when you are prepared to accept a longer working day, but leave work on time the rest of the week. If work is taking up more time than you like there may actually be nothing you can do about this – it is what you need to do to pay the mortgage. It is patronising to suggest that everyone can work the hours they want at no financial cost. This makes it all the more important to view each leisure hour as being worth more than gold, not something to be frittered away. Spend it on what *you* believe to be important. If it what you really enjoy doing, that time is never wasted.

● **Emotional stress.** This is a tough one as it is so broad. Basically, it involves being able to completely separate work from problems in your personal life. Think of your workplace as being 'safe' from your emotional turmoil and use a mental image to achieve this. While travelling to work, pick an arbitrary point on the way and imagine you are dropping off a bag with all your emotional problems in it. Because you have left these behind you are not allowed to think about them until you mentally pick that bag up again on the way home. You can then once again begin to deal with your personal problems, having had a rest from them. This may seem strange at first, but after a few days it will become automatic. Try it – it works.

I leave the last word to a patient of mine who died from cancer. Even in the advanced stages of his illness he focused on the business ideas he had always wanted to pursue, because, 'I only have one run at this world – it's not a dress rehearsal. The world will not change for me so I need to go out and change it. Doing that makes me feel really good.' I often remember those words as a guiding example of how to view life and stay content in the process. His age? Seventeen.

KEY POINTS

● Stress means many things to many people, but it usually involves change of some description.
● A major source of stress is anxiety about the unknown: what might occur rather than what is happening now.
● We all need stress to function properly but too much, over too long a time, can cause serious problems.
● Stress shows itself in many symptoms, both physical and mental.

- Stress is often made worse by excessive consumption of cigarettes and alcohol and a poor diet.
- Very often stress is a question of what pressures you allow yourself to be put under, particularly at work, and therefore much of the answer is in your hands.
- Keep a stress diary, look at this honestly and discuss it with your partner or a trusted friend, to work out where the sources of stress in your life lie.
- Use deep breathing and other relaxation techniques to prepare for situations that you find stressful, as well as practising these regularly to improve your general well-being.

12
SMOKING

'I have every sympathy with the American who was so horrified by what he read of the effects of smoking that he gave up reading.'
– **Lord Conesford**

If, as I lie on my deathbed, I'm asked what I've gleaned from my years on this earth, I suspect I will close my eyes and think for many long moments. I will then open them and, looking into the eyes of my nearest and dearest, mutter the immortal phrase, 'All men want to be James Bond.'

Actually most of the men I know, if pressed, have wanted to be James Bond at some point in their life and I was no exception. Sitting in the front row of my local cinema at an impressionable age, I remember the first time Sean Connery appeared on the screen, immaculately dressed in black tie and white dinner jacket and beating all comers at the casino. It is a defining first moment in the whole series of 007 films when he looks up after lighting a cigarette and through a cloud of smoke says, 'The name's Bond, James Bond.' According to Ian Fleming's original novel, Bond puffed his way through 70 high-tar, unfiltered cigarettes a day specially made for him from a blend of Macedonian tobacco, and yet in the films you never hear him cough once. In the real world, agent 007 would now be long dead, either from emphysema or lung cancer, and no sane man has the desire to follow him down that path. In fact, if you look at his lifestyle as a whole, if the lung cancer hadn't got him, the booze, sexually transmitted infections or his enemies' bullets should have killed him off by the end of the first book.

It is ironic that so many icons of cool in Hollywood history have succumbed to their habit of smoking. You only have to think of Humphrey Bogart, who was rarely seen without a cigarette in his hand, or Steve McQueen, to name but two, to realise how much talent has been cut short by the little white sticks.

Smokers turn off when a doctor goes on about the effects of smoking and I certainly try not to hammer my patients about it. However, if this habit, more than any other, ceased to exist, it would start both to improve the health of the whole nation and make my life a whole lot easier. Smoking causes 22% of all male deaths and at least 40% of smokers will die from smoking-related diseases. These include the obvious suspects, such as lung cancer, heart disease, strokes and chronic lung disease, but also cancers of the bladder, stomach, throat and mouth.

Every time a smoker lights up a cigarette, that cigarette is shortening their life by an average of about five minutes. I'm not going to dwell too long on the perils of smoking – you would have to be from Mars to argue that tobacco does not cause significant health problems – but instead I'm going to look at ways of giving up, which, in the end, is what it is all about. Men may start smoking to look cool, rebellious or even heroic, but, take it from me, there is nothing cool or heroic about dying from cancer as an emaciated skeleton. In any case, most smokers long to quit, as many studies have shown.

But why should smoking be so enjoyable in the first place?

Well, the cigarette is perhaps the finest drug-delivery system that has ever been invented. A smoker drawing on a cigarette will have chemicals hitting their brain as fast, if not faster, than if they had injected them into their arm. Nicotine is an immensely addictive drug, so much so that a few years ago the Surgeon General of the USA defined it as being as addictive as heroin. It provides the nervous system with an instant and intense stimulation that can be initially pleasurable and can reduce tiredness and anxiety.

Unfortunately, apart from being highly addictive, tobacco contains over 400 chemicals, including such delights as arsenic, cyanide, benzine and carbon monoxide. I must have heard every excuse from smokers as to why they haven't quite managed to quit, but unfortunately there are no alternatives to actually stopping. Cutting down is, in the long term, of little help as the addictive nature of nicotine means that even if you smoke only one or two cigarettes a day you are in a constant battle with the habit which you are unlikely to win however strong your willpower.

There is also little point in switching to low-tar cigarettes as these appear to be almost as dangerous as the higher-tar brands. In any case, smokers of low-tar brands often subconsciously either inhale more deeply or actually cover up the filter holes on the cigarette with their fingers to get the same hit of nicotine. It is ironic and ultimately depressing that some smokers of low-tar cigarettes are subject to particularly aggressive forms of tobacco-linked lung cancer.

STOPPING SMOKING

The many benefits of stopping smoking should be obvious, but let's look at the principal ones:

- Within 10–15 years of giving up, an ex-smoker's risk of developing lung cancer is only slightly greater than someone who has never smoked.
- You will gradually feel fitter and perform better in all walks of life, including in the bedroom (smoking can affect your erections and damage your sperm count).
- You won't smell like an ashtray, your teeth will not be yellow and you will actually be able to taste food again.
- Children of smokers are at higher risk of asthma, cot death, bronchitis and glue ear. Several hundred adults in the UK also die every year from breathing other people's cigarette smoke.
- In terms of cash, if you smoke 20 cigarettes a day you will send at least £1,000 a year up in smoke, and this figure continues to rise year after year.

Never mind the lecture, I hear you say, how do I stop smoking for good? First of all, you really do have to want to stop smoking, so I often say to patients that half-hearted in this situation actually means half-failed before you have even started. Begin by making a list of all the unpleasant aspects of smoking and put it in a prominent place in your house to remind you why you want to give up. Look at this every day. See if a friend or colleague will actually give up with you so that you have moral support and can lean on each other if things get tough.

Be prepared for a hard time for the first two or three weeks and then, if it happens, it will not come as a shock. However, it might not come to that and you may be pleasantly surprised, for some people do seem to stop completely painlessly and easily. Keep a smoking diary, noting when you light up and what is happening at the times you smoke. Many people find they smoke after eating or in response to stressful situations at work or elsewhere, and it is a good idea to work out other things to do at such times.

Some people like to choose a date to stop smoking completely and count down to it, cutting down slowly. But I've never known this gradual approach be very effective, and the evidence certainly is that it is less so than stopping altogether. The fact is, the more you cut down, the more important each cigarette seems to become and the harder it can be to give up the last one or two. When you quit, throw out ashtrays, lighters and any smoking-related paraphernalia and in the first week or two try to avoid other smokers. This may mean stopping at a time when you are away from work or are not under too much stress and have got other things to occupy yourself, such as when you are on holiday. Keep a large jar at home and every day put into it the money you would have spent on cigarettes and watch how quickly the pounds mount up. Promise yourself a treat and then go out and buy it with the money you have saved.

The unpalatable truth here is that it is ultimately down to you to succeed and this will only happen if – and here I must repeat – you really are ready to quit.

However, far more aids to stopping smoking are now available than ever before, and if you can accept that the urge to smoke will lessen and pass, these can be very helpful in getting you through the first few dangerous days. We'll consider these methods in a moment, but first why not give the Henderson Quit Plan a try? This very simple approach has been shown to work and can be summed up as follows:

● Practise the four Ds. *Deep* breathing will calm you down when you get the urge to light up. Slowly inhale and exhale as if you were taking the first drag on a cigarette. *Drink* water, the colder the better, throughout the day and whenever you crave a cigarette. *Do* something else when you want to smoke – whether it is going for a walk, digging a ditch or standing on your head. *Delay* reaching for a cigarette. Remember – the longer you put off giving in to the craving the nearer you get to being able to say you have quit.

- Rather than substituting chocolate bars or sweets for cigarettes, as many people do, try eating more fruit or carrots.
- Buy a stress ball to keep your hands busy instead of reaching for a cigarette. These can be squeezed, punched or even thrown at the wall.
- Consider joining a stop-smoking support group as this can make a significant difference to your chances of giving up if you feel weak-willed.

You may, though, prefer to go straight to one of the other methods I mentioned above. Even so, the tips I suggest are likely to be useful in your attempt to quit. Probably the most popular method is nicotine replacement therapy (NRT), which has been shown to double the chances of quitting compared with using willpower alone.

NICOTINE REPLACEMENT THERAPY

It is the nicotine in tobacco that makes people addicted to smoking, so when you stop smoking your body craves nicotine and it is this craving that makes you want to start smoking again. Various methods based on nicotine replacement have helped many smokers to quit and are available either on prescription or over the counter. The aim in each of these is to limit the withdrawal effects of stopping smoking while gradually reducing your body's nicotine level over time. Your body painlessly gets used to having less and less of the stimulant, until you are able to stop without it noticing.

The three types of NRT most often used in the UK are nicotine patches, nicotine gum and nicotine inhalators.

● **Nicotine patches.** These look like oversized plasters and are applied to the skin in a similar way. The patch contains nicotine which is slowly released into the body through the skin. However, you may still need to use willpower because NRT may not completely remove your desire to smoke.

For the first few weeks you use patches that contain a higher level of nicotine and then step down to ones containing less nicotine. Patches are available in forms that supply a constant dose of nicotine for 16 or 24 hours, but there is no evidence that a 24-hour patch is more effective, or that tapering off your use of patches is more effective than suddenly stopping them. Most people use nicotine patches for eight weeks, although this varies between individuals and according to the brand of patch. Nicotine from nicotine patches is absorbed at a much slower rate into the body than from a cigarette, and there is little evidence that people can become addicted to them. A further benefit is that this nicotine does not contain the other harmful chemicals released by cigarettes.

When using nicotine patches:

● Always apply a patch to a hairless, clean area of skin between the neck and the waist – for example, the upper arm, back or shoulder.

- Try to vary the site each day.
- Wear each patch all day. Do not remove it to smoke a cigarette, as some people do!

Combining nicotine patches with other forms of nicotine replacement therapy may be more effective than using patches alone. Moreover, it appears to be just as safe, although relatively little research has been conducted on this as yet. Standard-strength patches have been found to be more effective than lower-dose patches in medium to heavy smokers (more than 10 cigarettes a day).

Nicotine patches are safe for most people. However, because nicotine can increase the heart rate and blood pressure, people with a history of heart attack or serious heart problems, such as angina or irregular heartbeats, should take care when using them. If you are in any of these categories, consult your doctor before using this therapy.

The main side effect from using nicotine patches is the possibility of a skin rash developing at the location of the patch. For this reason people with sensitive skin or multiple allergies may find patches unsuitable. Applying the new patch to a different part of the body each day can help, as can simple antihistamine creams.

Other possible side effects include sleep disturbances or insomnia (removing the patch after 9pm each evening may help here), vivid dreams and nausea. The advantages of patches are that they are simple to use, effective, provide a steady supply of nicotine and the different strengths allow them to be tailored to the individual smoker's needs. Patches are also discreet, as they can easily be hidden from sight under clothing. Their disadvantages include possible skin irritation and allergic reactions, there is little benefit in using them for more than eight weeks and you may be tempted to smoke despite using them.

● **Nicotine gum.** This form of NRT can also double your chances of stopping smoking compared to relying on willpower alone. It looks like chewing gum and contains a nicotine compound (nicotine polacrilex) designed to slowly release nicotine into the mouth when chewed and then placed between the cheek and gum. Nicotine gum is available without a prescription and in various strengths.

One piece of nicotine gum is chewed slowly for approximately 30 minutes whenever you have the urge to smoke. For highly dependent smokers (more than 20 cigarettes a day), a starting dose of 4 milligrams of gum is more effective than one of 2 milligrams. As with patches, you may still need to use willpower as well because nicotine gum alone may not completely remove the desire to smoke.

Do not use more than 15 pieces of gum in 24 hours and always chew the gum correctly – if you swallow it the nicotine is wasted. Chew the gum slowly until the taste becomes strong, then stop chewing and rest the gum against the inside of your cheek. When the taste starts to fade, start chewing again until the taste becomes strong once more, then rest the gum again. Keep chewing and resting the gum for about half an hour per piece, by which time the gum will no longer have any taste. Dispose of the gum hygienically. Repeat the procedure again the next time you want to smoke.

Avoid eating or drinking for 15 minutes before using the gum and do not eat or drink while chewing, because some beverages can reduce its effectiveness. Do not smoke while using nicotine replacement, otherwise you risk unpleasant side effects as a result of the body getting too much nicotine.

Using nicotine gum may produce these common side effects:

- Your tongue may tingle while chewing.
- You may get hiccups.
- You may develop mouth ulcers, or a sore mouth.
- You may have some indigestion — chewing the gum incorrectly and not 'parking' it between your cheek and gum sometimes causes this.
- Chewing can cause jaw pain. If you have problems with your jaw joint (temperomandibular or TMJ disorders), nicotine gum may not be for you.
- You may not like the taste of some nicotine gums. Mint and citrus flavours are available and many people prefer these to plain gum.

To sum up, nicotine gum is simple to use, many people find the idea of chewing gum familiar and very acceptable, gum provides a steady supply of nicotine, the choice of different strengths means that the needs of each user can be met and, finally, you can readily check how much gum you are using each day. On the minus side, some people do not like the taste, you may not want to be seen chewing gum in public and you may still be tempted to smoke.

- **Nicotine inhalator.** Also sometimes called a nicotine inhaler, this looks very much like a cigarette but is not actually smoked. It holds a cartridge containing nicotine which you use to deliver a puff of nicotine vapour (in a measured dose) whenever you feel a craving for a cigarette.

Absorbed into your mouth and throat, this helps you to overcome any of the effects of no longer receiving nicotine from cigarettes.

There is little hard evidence that one form of NRT is more effective than another, but some people want to replace the act of smoking with an activity that feels similar and for this reason they prefer to use a nicotine inhalator. Here again you are taking nicotine in a 'clean' form and you are twice as likely to stay cigarette-free as you are by relying on just willpower.

Whenever you feel the urge to have a cigarette, put a nicotine cartridge into the inhalator and suck hard on the mouthpiece until you can taste the nicotine. Keep sucking on the inhalator until there is no more taste. For most people a cartridge gives about 20 minutes of heavy use. On average about six cartridges a day are used, but you should never use more than 12. In cold weather you may find that you have to work harder to get the same amount of nicotine from the inhalator than you do on warmer days. The mouthpiece should be cleaned several times a week by rinsing it in water for hygiene purposes.

Nicotine inhalators are safe for most people, but if you have heart disease consult your doctor before using this therapy.

You may experience a slightly sore mouth or gums when using an inhalator, especially if the maximum recommended number of cartridges is used each day. However, they are simple to use and their effectiveness may be enhanced in people who prefer to use a cigarette substitute, rather than nicotine patches or gum.

Apart from NRT, there are various other ways to stop smoking:

WILLPOWER

This is the simplest method – you simply stop smoking and decide not to start again. However much you may want a cigarette, you say to yourself that you can and will resist the temptation, and simply do not have one. It is purely strength of will that stops you from picking up a cigarette, even though you may be experiencing some of the classic side effects of nicotine withdrawal, such as irritability, insomnia and sweating.

Much depends on how motivated you are to stop. Most smokers do not continue to smoke from choice but because they are addicted to nicotine. You are not alone – 70% of smokers in the UK would like to quit and every year three million of them try to.

No chemicals or drugs are used to reinforce willpower and so this is the safest and simplest form of stopping smoking there is. In addition, willpower costs nothing, it does not involve any drugs or nicotine substitutes and, of course, there are no side effects unless you count the nicotine withdrawal symptoms that you must combat. On the negative side, it has been shown that if 100 people choose to stop smoking at the same time using willpower alone, only three of them will still be cigarette-free one year later.

HYPNOTHERAPY

Hypnotherapy creates a state of deep mental relaxation in which physical and mental stress and tension are reduced. Someone in this state of mind may be more open to suggestions from a professionally trained hypnotherapist about how to change certain aspects of their behaviour or lifestyle – such as smoking. Hypnotherapy has been widely promoted for many years as an effective way of helping smokers to quit and is said to strengthen the will to stop. However, a major analysis of nine controlled studies I looked at found that it did not have a greater effect on quit rates after six months than either other treatments or willpower alone.

Almost anyone who wishes to be hypnotised – willingness is essential here – can achieve a level of relaxation sufficient to allow it to take place. During the experience, which is usually a pleasant one, you are aware of your surroundings and can come out of the hypnotised state at any time. There are only a few medical conditions that do not allow hypnotherapy to be carried out, no nicotine replacement or drugs are involved and there are few obvious side effects. On the other hand, hypnotherapy does not appear to be effective in helping smokers to kick the habit, and it can be expensive.

ACUPUNCTURE

Acupuncture is a traditional form of alternative treatment for a wide range of illnesses. Originating in the Far East thousands of years ago, it aims to improve the overall well-being of the patient, rather than treat specific symptoms in isolation. According to traditional Chinese philosophy, our health is dependent on the body's motivating energy, or qi (pronounced 'kee'), moving in a smooth and balanced way through a series of meridians (channels) beneath the skin. Qi consists of equal and opposite qualities – yin and yang – and when these become unbalanced, illness may result. By inserting fine needles into the channels of energy, an acupuncturist can stimulate the body's own healing response and help to restore its natural balance. The flow of qi can be disturbed by a number of factors. These include emotional states such as anxiety, stress, anger, fear or grief, poor nutrition, weather conditions, hereditary factors, infections, poisons and trauma.

On the basis that it is claimed to reduce nicotine withdrawal symptoms, acupuncture has long been promoted as a successful aid in helping smokers to quit. However, when compared with other anti-smoking treatments in a wide range of scientific studies, acupuncture appears to be less effective. Incidentally, the same caveat appears to apply to laser therapy and electro-stimulation.

Acupuncture seems to be safe when performed by an experienced practitioner, but should you consider trying it, always make sure that the practitioner concerned is registered with the British Acupuncture Council.

There may be some temporary local discomfort in some areas when an acupuncture needle is inserted, but this is transient and there are no other regularly reported side effects. Acupuncture remains a popular alternative to other methods for smokers who prefer a 'natural' method of trying to quit.

NON-NICOTINE-BASED DRUG TREATMENTS

These are drug treatments that may help people to stop smoking. Clonidine, used to treat high blood pressure, has been shown to be effective, although it can have significant side effects. There are studies that show that mecamylamine – when used in combination with nicotine replacement therapy – can aid smoking cessation.

There are two reasons why anxiolytic (anti-anxiety) drugs may help you stop smoking. Firstly, they can reduce the anxiety that sometimes occurs during nicotine withdrawal. Secondly, smoking addiction appears to be partly due to deficits in the brain chemicals dopamine, serotonin and norepinephrine, all of which are increased in quantity by anxiolytic drugs.

Evidence is growing that antidepressants may also be beneficial in helping smokers to give up the habit. The reason for this is unclear, but it could be that because depression is sometimes a symptom of nicotine withdrawal, and because stopping the comforting ritual of smoking may itself trigger depression, antidepressants can help smokers to quit. Also, nicotine may have an antidepressant effect on some smokers, making it even more difficult for them to stop, and this is perhaps why antidepressants can help. However, I rarely suggest this type of treatment, preferring, if I prescribe anything here, to suggest Zyban.

A prescription-only medicine originally designed as an antidepressant, Zyban (buproprion) is a classic example of the role of serendipity in medicine. Although the drug was not very effective as an antidepressant, it was quickly realised that people taking it lost their desire to smoke and nearly a decade on it helps about one in three of those who take it to give up smoking. Zyban does not contain nicotine but instead works by affecting the centres in the brain known to be associated with addiction, and by increasing the amount of the chemicals dopamine and noradrenaline there. It is thought that in doing so it reproduces the effects of the nicotine in tobacco and so reduces the need to smoke. As a bonus it seems to damp down the typical physical symptoms of nicotine withdrawal and may help prevent significant weight gain at this time, although this aspect of its use is still being researched.

Bupropion was tested in two clinical trials, published in the *New England Journal of Medicine*, which showed that 30% of users did not smoke one year after treatment. The comparable figure for people using NRT is 16%.

Before we all go rushing to the doctor to obtain this wonder drug, a word or two of caution. It is best used in the context of an intensive smoking cessation support strategy, and there has been adverse media publicity regarding the death of patients recently starting Zyban. However, these deaths have mainly been due to diseases associated with smoking or linked to incorrect prescribing of the drug. Zyban is a prescription-only medicine, and typically lasts for seven weeks, depending on when the user feels capable of managing without further help. On the first three days the patient takes one tablet daily, and from the fourth day two tablets are taken daily at intervals of at least eight hours. It takes one week for Zyban to have its maximum effect and so I recommend my patients start taking it one to two weeks before they stop smoking.

Possible side effects include sleeping problems, agitation, anxiety, dryness of the mouth, skin rashes and headache. More serious side effects are fits, which affect approximately one patient in 1,000 taking Zyban, so people who suffer from epilepsy must not use the drug. Nor must those with eating disorders such as bulimia and anorexia.

Whatever option they use to help them stop smoking, I often recommend my patients in the UK to phone the NHS Smoking Helpline which is an excellent source of advice on all aspects of smoking and giving up. Specialist advisers are available to discuss problems or give advice and the lines are open daily.

KEY POINTS

- Smoking is the single biggest cause of preventable death in the UK.
- There is no such thing as a 'safer' cigarette.
- There are a number of ways in which smokers can be helped provided they genuinely wish to quit. These include nicotine replacement therapy (NRT) and drug treatments.
- All methods require determination – there is no magic cure for nicotine addiction.
- Most doctors run stop-smoking clinics at their surgeries.

13
NATURAL TREATMENTS

'First, do no harm.'
– Hippocrates

Being the sort of chap who is really most comfortable in a three-piece suit and who starches his upper lip before breakfast, I'm hardly someone who would readily be labelled an ageing hippie. However, many years as a GP have rounded away the sharp edges of conventional scientific dogma and made me realise that there are far more ways of treating someone than with a prescription.

One of these is, of course, time and we are very fortunate as family doctors in that the majority of illnesses we see are, in fact, self-limiting and will get better irrespective of what we do to our patients. This is just as well, otherwise the NHS would grind to a halt within a week. Another is simply allowing the patient to talk their problems through. This can be a powerful tool in helping them feel better and overcome a physical or psychological bottleneck, which, once released, allows them to naturally improve once more. It is this ability to let someone unburden themselves, I believe, that under-lies the success of many of the natural treatments that have multiplied over the past decade. The one thread which runs through all complementary therapies is that they allow the patient to talk at length about what is bothering them. I'm convinced that this is the pivotal aspect of each of these treatments, and that it aids recovery in the long term. At the same time this realisation brings home to me the frustrations of running surgeries in the NHS. I spend an average of only seven or eight minutes with each patient and simply don't have the time to discuss issues in as much detail as I would like.

Be that as it may, over the years I've recommended a number of natural supplements to my patients which seem to come up with the goods time and time again. For me these products have enough scientific evidence behind them to allow me to recommend them, and above all they are safe. On the other hand, out there in the natural supplements market there is an inordinate amount of junk which does absolutely nothing for my patients but which makes some producers very rich. Sorting the wheat from the chaff can be a very time-consuming and frustrating exercise. I do not believe you need to be some supplement freak to gain benefit from a handful of supplements, although I must emphasise that they are no replacement for a well-rounded lifestyle that includes a healthy diet and a positive mental attitude.

NATURAL SUPPLEMENTS THAT WORK

In no particular order the natural supplements that I recommend most often are:

● **Glucosamine.** This is one of the natural supplements most acceptable to the medical community. I realised this about a year ago when I received a letter from a hard-nosed orthopaedic consultant asking me to start one of my arthritic patients on it. Surgeons are not usually known for their benign attitude towards non-conventional medicine. (How do you confuse a surgeon? Ask him for the names of two antibiotics.) So there really must be something going on if glucosamine has permeated to the higher echelons of consultant prescribing. It is perhaps now the most widely used supplement for those seeking relief from painful joints and inflamed tissue and its success appears to be linked to its being a natural component of cartilage. It has been found to stimulate cartilage cells to synthesise production of the chemicals that help to lubricate our joints, and although we produce glucosamine ourselves to some degree, this production capacity lessens as we age and over the age of 50 we start to significantly run into the red.

There have been significant studies performed on glucosamine that have compared the disease symptoms in arthritic patients, as measured by X-rays, between those taking a daily dose of glucosamine and those taking simple sugar pills. The X-rays of those taking the sugar pills continued to worsen while in patients taking glucosamine they revealed no evidence of a worsening of the symptoms. These studies also found that patients on glucosamine have less pain and stiffness than those taking a placebo drug and that glucosamine appears to have a low incidence of side effects, the commonest being either mild diarrhoea or indigestion in about 1% of patients. I take glucosamine for my back (when I remember to) and have found it to be very effective.

The recommended dose is important here and should be 1,500 milligrams of glucosamine sulphate per day. Note that I say glucosamine sulphate, because various preparations on the market are jumping on this particular bandwagon, and it was glucosamine sulphate that was studied in the scientific trials. It must also be remembered that any improvement will not happen overnight but will take six to eight weeks to become significant. All joints appear to benefit, but knee and hip joints probably do so most.

● **CoEnzyme Q10 (CoQ10).** I must confess that I had not heard of this supplement until some years ago, but having been recommending it to patients who are either fatigued or suffering from post-viral lethargy, I've no doubt that it can work and work well. This is basically an antioxidant which is found in every cell of our bodies and which helps with the cellular production of energy. Now popular with high-level non-doping athletes and Olympians, it helps boost the body's defences as well as promoting the oxidation of its tissues. If you are fortunate enough to be able to have a diet rich in raw foods, as well as tuna and oily fish, spinach and pulses, you are probably getting enough CoQ10 each day. However, because cooking and processing often destroy it, supplementation may be needed, and if you are generally feeling fatigued my usual starting recommendation is 30 milligrams twice a day. Interestingly, levels of CoQ10 have been shown to be low in men suffering from heart disease, and I've yet to hear of any side effects in a heart patient taking it or indeed any side effects at all.

● **St John's Wort.** This herb, also known as hypericum, hit the headlines in the *British Medical Journal* in 1996 when it was reported to be a promising treatment for depression. Extracts of hypericum were shown to be significantly superior to dummy pills and as effective as standard anti-depressants. In addition, it was reported at that time that the herb might offer an advantage over antidepressants in terms of tolerability, which could improve patient compliance.

St John's Wort is a short, yellow-flowered plant that was described by Hippocrates, the father of medicine, and so has been used medicinally for thousands of years. For some reason the Germans seem to love St John's Wort and in that country over half of all cases of depression, anxiety and insomnia are treated with it, with antidepressants such as Prozac being used for only 2%. Figures in the UK are very different, but there is no doubt that more and more people are taking the drug to treat stress and stress-related problems. Just to show how potent this treatment can be, it has just been licensed in the UK as a prescription drug and under EC guidelines more and more countries are going down this route.

Stressed men and men over the age of 50 who are going through a mid-life crisis or moving dangerously close to clinical depression may benefit from taking St John's Wort. The optimum dose, based on the majority of medical studies, is 300 milligrams three times a day and most over-the-counter preparations now come in this form. At least six weeks at this dosage is required to eat into any kind of mild depression and so you should not give up if you are not feeling better after only a week or two. Also, you should resist the temptation to take more, thinking that more is better — it is not. Like prescription antidepressants, St John's Wort is not addictive, a stimulant or an energy booster. Unlike many prescription antidepressants, its side effects are few and its extensive use in Europe has not resulted in any medical reports of serious drug interactions. Reported side effects tend to be very mild indeed, with about 0.5% of patients saying that they felt more tired or had mild stomach upset. Some studies have reported a slightly higher incidence of side effects, but I virtually never see problems when giving this drug to men. Contrast this with the fact that about a third of all people taking conventional antidepressants report significant or disabling side effects and you can see how beneficial St John's Wort can be in selected patients.

● **Echinacea.** Now the top-selling herb in the USA, echinacea, commonly known as purple cone flower, was originally a North American Indian remedy. Because it appears to be beneficial in treating problems stemming from an under-functioning immune system, I sometimes recommend it to help fight off colds and flu. It is believed to work by increasing the activity and concentration of white blood cells in the body as well as helping to boost production of interferon. This is critical in keeping the body's defences in top shape and some of my patients swear that taking the drug is the reason why they don't get colds. Echinacea can also be useful in ear and sinus infections, and in helping to prevent sore throats and cystitis.

The drug has an interesting property in that, if it is taken all the time, its effects seem to wear off. For this reason you need to take regular breaks from it or it will have no benefit. I usually suggest that my patients take it for a month at a time and then have a two- or three-week break before starting it again for another month. As men age it becomes increasingly important that they do not suffer from recurring colds or flu-like illnesses, and echinacea can be a safe and simple way of helping them to do so.

● **Multivitamins.** A slightly contentious one this, since there is no doubt that a wide and balanced daily input of vitamins is crucial to long-term health. But how much is too much, and which vitamins do we need to supplement anyway? If you are following a sensible eating plan (see the chapter Diet and Weight), vitamin supplementation will probably not be needed. However, men over the age of 50 can require extra vitamins, especially if they are unwell, smoke or eat irregularly. But, rather than take mega-doses of vitamins, my advice to patients is to make sure they are having a multivitamin supplement that has 100% of the recommended daily intake of each vitamin. (These amounts are now shown on all labels of vitamin products.) I regard this as the best general approach to supplementation, but if I were to recommend particular vitamins, it would be vitamin C at a daily dose of at least 500 milligrams, as this may help beat a cold and boost immunity.

The theory behind this goes back some 30 years, to when the American Nobel Laureate Linus Pauling created a major stir in the medical community by claiming that vitamin C, when taken in huge doses, could reduce or stop the symptoms of a cold. This notion is still hotly debated in many quarters, but what seems to happen here is that the symptoms we all know when we get a cold are probably little to do with the cold virus itself but more to do with the body's own response to this alien invader. During a cold the fine membranes that line our nose become very rich in white blood cells designed to fight off the cold virus. The trouble is, they can also contribute to inflammation of these membranes and so worsen the runny nose so familiar to us all. The use of large amounts of vitamin C is therefore a two-pronged attack, with the first prong giving support to our own immune system and the second minimising how our body attacks itself when we have a cold.

Like many doctors, I don't seem to get many colds because my patients sitting in front of me sneezing into my face expose me to a constant sub-clinical attack from viruses all year round. But if I did feel the need to protect myself, vitamin C would probably be my starting point.

● **Lycopene.** This is the red pigment found in tomatoes, which has been implicated as being protective against prostate cancer. Trials of men suffering from this problem showed that those who had received 15 milligrams of lycopene each day had smaller tumours than those who had not been taking it. In another study of 48,000 American men it was found that consumption of tomato products more than twice weekly, as opposed to never, was linked to a 34% reduction in risk.

It is not only the prostate gland that may benefit here – there is also evidence that people on a cooked-tomato-rich diet have a reduced risk of heart disease. In one study of people from ten European countries, those on a diet rich in lycopene had about half the rate of heart attacks of those not on one. Pre-boiled tomato juice has also been implicated in protecting the body's cells against damage caused by cigarette smoke.

The average amount of lycopene the body can absorb varies from 3 milligrams to 7 milligrams a day, depending on body size. For existing prostate problems, 10 milligrams is the recommended daily dose, and to protect against prostate disease try 5 milligrams daily. (To get this second amount, try grilling four or five average-sized tomatoes, since cooking releases five times more lycopene than is available from raw tomatoes.)

Lycopene is thought to work by neutralising naturally occurring cell-damaging molecules – our old friends free radicals – produced by the body in response to air pollution and smoke inhalation. The possibility that many of us are exposed to more free radicals in the environment than the body can deactivate has led to the belief that these are implicated in the onset and development of many degenerative diseases.

DO NATURAL TREATMENTS WORK?

I'm often asked about natural treatments for men. Of course, most of these therapies are intended for either sex, but the problem here is that there are now so many that I could fill this book just discussing the first few in detail. The ones that patients discuss with me now almost daily include homeopathy, Reiki and reflexology. Homeopathy, which is extremely popular, brings to mind the central tenet of all medicine, dating as far back as Hippocrates – 'Firstly, do no harm.' When discussing homeopathy, and alternative medicine in general, we should perhaps be thinking not 'Will it harm?' but rather 'Will it work?' Until recently any medical student would work through their training years with little or no mention of any non-conventional treatments and if any were discussed it was usually with a cynical smile from a teaching professor hostile to the whole idea.

However, a recent study undertaken to find out what support there would be among GPs for a homeopathic service found that only 10% of GPs who responded had never recommended or referred patients for any complementary therapy, while the majority had actually suggested homeopathy to a patient at some time. Not only that, but half the GPs wanted further training in complementary therapy in order to broaden their working knowledge of this area of medicine. Many similar studies have suggested that there is a much greater desire among doctors to learn more about homeopathy and other forms of natural treatment than there was just 20 years ago.

So far so good, but nothing is ever this simple, and homeopathy is no exception. There is a juggernaut-sized fly in this particular ointment and it takes the shape of scientific analysis. To understand why conventional medicine, while becoming more open-minded in many quarters, remains to be won over by homeopathy, we must first look at why it is said to work in the first place. It is a system that revolves around the theory that 'like cures like', so that a poison that is causing symptoms of an illness in an individual can be used to treat those same symptoms. The body is believed by homeopaths to be integrated by a 'vital force' that maintains its normal healthy functioning and that illness occurs when this force is put under strain. Symptoms of illness are viewed as the body healing itself by using its own natural powers, and homeopathy aims to stimulate this self-healing process. Substances are diluted many times – to the point where virtually no molecules of the original substance remain – and administered by homeopaths in the belief that these preparations retain sufficient 'likeness' to the illness to stimulate self-healing by the body.

From the point of view of the medical establishment, this is where the wheels start to come off the homeopathic wagon. While many doctors accept that small quantities of a chemical substance can alter physiological activity in the body, it is hard to see the logic in using a substance so diluted that it is said to be the equivalent of a pinch of salt in the Atlantic Ocean. The theory that electromagnetic 'footprints' of the original substance remain in the diluted mixture, to which the body then responds – the so-called 'water memory' theory – is viewed as risible and completely against all the laws of science by most medical experts. Many doctors feel that any beneficial effects of homeopathy that are described are due in part to a combination of the placebo effect of taking any medication – conventional or alternative – and the considerable time given by homeopathic practitioners to their clients. Consultations of an hour or more may take place, during which close attention is paid to factors such as emotions and the personal beliefs of that individual. This is something that many NHS doctors know can be of immense benefit to their patients but which they are simply unable to provide within the current constraints of the health service.

So, does homeopathy appear to be of benefit to some patients whom conventional medicine seems unable to help? Undoubtedly. Are doctors as a group slowly recognising that many patients now view homeopathy and other 'natural' treatments as their initial preferred option? Probably. Is there any logical basis in science why homeopathy should work and that a 'vital force' holds our health and well-being together? Not a shred.

What about acupuncture? many patients ask me. This has been practised for many thousands of years in the Far East but has taken hold in the West since the 1970s, especially after an article published in the *New York Times* by a journalist who enthusiastically wrote of its pain-relieving properties following removal of his appendix. In the UK there are now two main forms of acupuncture. The first is the traditional Chinese form, practitioners of which believe that illness arises from an imbalance of the life forces known as yin and yang, and insert needles into various body points to try to restore the balance.

The second form is more widely practised and is based on the physical effects a needle can have on the body. Needles are inserted into 'trigger points', known as acupoints – sensitive points that are often at areas where nerves enter or leave muscle and tissue. The theory is that if you put a needle into such a trigger point, natural endorphin painkillers are released into the bloodstream, as well as natural anti-inflammatory compounds that promote healing.

Acupuncture has many converts who claim it helps all manner of ills, including back pain – and pain with virtually any cause, come to that – anxiety and stress, high blood pressure and irritable bowel problems, to name but a few. Hard scientific evidence is scarce here, although one study published in the *Journal of the Royal Society of Medicine* showed that stimulating an acupoint just above the wrist could eliminate nausea in pregnancy, and this work has been successfully reproduced since. Other studies have shown that acupuncture can reduce pain and nausea after surgery, and many doctors now take the view that it makes certain nerves work better by stimulating them. Interestingly, these nerves coincide with traditional Chinese acupoints.

I've even tried acupuncture myself. Why, you may ask, since I'm clearly sceptical about it. Well, for one thing the practitioner was my wife. The second was that I was curious. And the third was the fact that I was in significant discomfort from a neck problem that seemed resistant to my conventional treatments. There was surprisingly little discomfort apart from in those areas where I was having pain anyway, but when I looked at my neck and back in a mirror during the treatment I was amazed to see massive reddening around these places but nowhere else. This was apparently consistent with what was expected and I toddled off needle-less and happily cynical.

The next day I had no neck pain and have not suffered from this problem since. All in the mind? I think not. If ever there was a man determined to disprove acupuncture it was I and although this is hardly a scientific trial it does make you think, doesn't it?

My personal favourite natural treatment is Pilates, although I must confess I'm hardly a regular advocate of it. In fact, although I know all of the theory, most of the time my Pilates exercises involve turning the pages of a book on the subject. Be that as it may, this is an extremely beneficial way of improving strength and flexibility in men of all ages, especially men over 50, and of helping to keep the waist to a respectable size.

Ignoring the cult of celebrity that has attached itself to Pilates, with all the usual spin-offs of books, DVDs and breathless chat-show interviews, I like this form of therapy as it allows for slow and safe controlled movements that reduce the risk of injury. Based around a core principle of developing strong lower-back and abdominal muscles, Pilates is an extensive set of exercises designed to build muscle tone, strength and suppleness without adding lots of muscle bulk to the body. It is also an extremely good antidote to stress and is effective for people with back problems (such as myself) who have to be careful about what sort of exercise they do. It can be done at home, in classes or with a teacher or video, and a good workout can be achieved in 20–40 minutes. Also, you are never too old to try it!

Yoga is more popular with women than men and is essentially a system of body postures, stretching and breath-ing exercises. The therapeutic benefits of yoga have been accepted by the medical community for many years. In the UK it tends to be practised by athletes and as part of fitness regimes more for its ability to increase suppleness and reduce stress levels than for its full spiritual benefits. The twisting and postural exercises are often of use in any warm-up programme and reduce the chances of muscle pulls and strains. Yoga can also improve and encourage restful sleep, and a beneficial workout need last no more than 30 minutes.

The Alexander technique is an excellent adjunct to yoga and other stretching exercises as it improves posture and suppleness by retraining the body to stand correctly without strain or slouching. I have no doubt at all that it can help people with chronic back pain or shoulder and neck tension. Initially it is taught by a specialist teacher on a one-to-one basis. The teacher assesses the posture that you have adopted over many years of sitting and standing incorrectly and then follows the main maxim of the Alexander technique – 'Free the neck; let the neck go forward and upward; let the back lengthen and widen.' This practice becomes second nature after some time (this varies from person to person), so that any other exercise you undertake will have the advantage of being performed in a natural and stress-free posture.

Osteopathy is especially good in treating some sports injuries and problems of the repetitive strain type. It is based on the premise that all disease is based on the body's musculo-skeletal framework. Osteopaths aim to improve joint mobility as well as that of the soft tissues by a combination of massage and manipulation. After this there may be some muscular tenderness and exercise is best avoided for a day or two. Osteopathy should be avoided if there is a history of disc prolapse in the back, but this treatment can be very effective in 'freeing up' stiff joints or areas of muscle spasm caused by repetitive forms of exercise.

I recommend chiropractors quite often, and the difference between chiropractic and osteopathy is that the first is based on the principle that the spine is the main 'highway' between the body and brain and any misalignment here causes significant pain and stiffness elsewhere. Of all the natural treatments mentioned here, chiropractic has possibly the greatest body of medical evidence in its favour and it is recommended in the UK as part of the best treatment of low-back pain. In connection with sport and exercise it is useful in curing low-grade, long-term back and neck spasm and discomfort. The treatment can involve standard medical tests such as X-rays and blood pressure monitoring.

Whatever supplement or natural treatment you feel fits the bill for you, always take time to find out as much as you can about it, remember that more is not better, and use it as an adjunct to a generally healthy lifestyle rather than as a replacement for this.

KEY POINTS

- Natural supplements can be very effective if used correctly. However, many have not been proven to be of any use.
- Rather than taking a wide range of supplements, use only a carefully selected few, and then only if warranted.
- A healthy diet and a healthy lifestyle are the best supplements of all.
- Natural treatments vary greatly in their effectiveness, but nearly all have the benefit that they allow the patient time to relax and talk.

14

DIET AND WEIGHT

'Never eat more than you can lift.'
– **Miss Piggy**, *The Muppet Show*

I mentioned earlier in this book that obesity is fast becoming the major curse of the NHS. But it is not so much part of a trend as a sad fact of life that men over the age of 50 burn several hundred calories a day less to maintain a stable weight than they were doing in their thirties. It can be an increasing struggle to keep weight off as we age and this is one of the reasons why middle-aged spread can start to appear well before we reach 50 and is certainly a frequent problem after this age. To lose weight you need to either reduce your food intake or increase your activity or – best of all – do both.

But why lose weight in the first place? Well, the reasons are wide and many but, in a nutshell, you're not only likely to live longer but you will do so in better health. At my weight (11½ stone) and height (5ft 10in), I'm 30% less likely to die in any given year than if I weighed over 16 stone. I'm also some seven or eight times less likely to develop diabetes if I remain slim rather than become obese. In addition, a 20% increase in body weight causes a staggering 80% increase in the risk of heart disease.

There are also many other reasons why staying trim is

good for you, some of which may not be immediately obvious:

- You will reduce your risk of arthritis, bowel cancer and gallstones.
- You will have more energy simply through carrying less weight around.
- You will snore less and be less prone to problems such as obstructive sleep apnoea – a major cause of road accidents owing to men falling asleep at the wheel.
- Sex may improve. As you lose weight the levels of testosterone in the body rise, and as a result libido increases. Some men even say their penis looks longer since abdominal fat can make it appear to shorten by one or two inches.
- Self-confidence and self-esteem often increase.

I remember, as a medical student, doing ward rounds with an eminent professor who looked frankly cadaverous and whose ascetic regime was held in awe by most of us, although when push came to shove we basically thought he was nuts. I still remember him poking and prodding obese patients before leaning over and whispering to them that he wanted to see them again in six months, by which time he expected them to have lost a minimum of three stones. He would then cut short the usual protest with a glare and the words, 'Remember that no obese people came out of concentration camps.'

Thinking about this still makes me squirm, but there is some truth in the professor's crass statement. In fact, all the studies I've looked at have shown that, to put it simply, overweight people not only eat more than thin people but also burn up their food faster. This apparent paradox arises simply because the greater the body weight, the more that body consumes energy, and in this simple truth is the basic rationale of the whole dieting industry. Think about the last time you dieted. You cut down on how much you were eating, the weight starts to come off, but as you lose this you start to burn off fewer calories in a normal day. So, unless you increase your exercise regime (or start one) you will not only tend to stick at a certain weight but will feel hungry all the time despite eating less. The natural habit is, therefore, to eat because you are hungry, with the result that the pounds go back on (and often a few more on top) and you end up swearing never to diet again or feeling a complete failure, or both. To me, this cycle goes some way to explaining why we spend at least £1 billion a year on diets. It is also clear that at least 90% of slimmers have regained all the weight they may have lost during their diet within a year of starting it.

Now, can you guess the punchline? That's right – dieting alone is essentially doomed to fail for the vast majority of people. We have to exercise as well as changing our eating patterns if we are to lose weight consistently and keep that weight off. As a nation we are increasingly sedentary in both work and leisure activities, and one of my favourite statistics is that the average person in the UK spends about four hours a day watching television. Multiply that by seven days a week and you get twenty-eight hours. If, instead of sitting on front of the box, you had gone walking, done some simple exercise, had sex or even done some gardening, you would have burned off over 4,000 calories a week. This is nearly the equivalent of two days' food, and all because we sit on our backsides watching TV.

HOW OVERWEIGHT ARE YOU?

Since you're reading this chapter, I take it you're concerned about your weight. But do you know how much you should be aiming to shed? Rather than use the usual 'if my belt's too tight I need to lose a few pounds' method, try the two main scientific ways:

● **Body mass index (BMI).** Now often used by doctors rather than weight measurement alone, this is a way of assessing whether you are the right weight for your height. To do this, using metric values, you divide your weight by the square of your height. This might sound complicated but in fact it's very easy. If you are, say, 1.78 metres tall and weigh 78 kilograms, the calculation is 78 divided by 1.78 x 1.78 i.e. 3.2, which means your BMI is 24.4. You are aiming for a BMI of between 20 and 25 (22 is probably ideal), as under 20 is underweight, over 25 is overweight and over 30 is obese. The only slight drawback to this way of calculating healthy weight is that if you are a very fit athlete carrying a significant amount of muscle, you can have an apparently unhealthy BMI yet be very healthy overall. However, there are other possible measurements, such as:

● **The 'beer belly' test.** A simple measurement of your waist circumference, this is taken at a line around your natural waist – a point between the top of the hip bone and the bottom rib. Without cheating (for example, breathing in), place a tape measure all the way around your waist and check the measurement. If the result is between 37 and 39 inches you are overweight, but if you are 40 inches and above you are obese and need to shift some weight fast.

A variation on this test is to measure your hips at their widest part, again in inches. Divide your waist measurement by this measurement and if the ratio is greater than 0.95 you are getting fat and need to lose weight. In some ways this is a more useful test as it allows for an estimate of how much weight you are carrying around your waist compared with on your hips – the more on the waist the greater the health risk.

I once thought about writing a diet book but became slightly depressed when I went into my local book shop and saw how the shelves were already groaning under the weight of such books, with dozens more being added to their ranks every month. However, you do not have to be a rocket scientist to work out that a good diet is essentially one in which the food you eat contains all the essential nutrients needed by our bodies to promote not only physical but also mental health.

A BALANCED DIET

Ideally, there are three food groups that your diet should contain as a balanced mix. The first is protein, such as provided by meat, dairy produce, fish, eggs and pulses. This should make up about 15% of your daily diet.

Next come carbohydrates, such as found in bread, rice, potatoes, pasta and fruit, vegetables and salads. These should be the bulk of your diet, making up about 60% of your daily intake. As far as fruit and vegetables are concerned, you should eat a total of five portions a day.

Finally, there is fat, which should make up a maximum of 30% of your diet. This is where much of our problems arise as we tend to consume far too many high-fat, sugar-rich, processed foods as well as eating the wrong sort of fats, such as lard and butter. Vegetable oils are much better for you and you can remember which, along with these, are the 'good' types of fat by using a simple little formula: at room temperature, fats that are liquid are better than fats that are solid. Liquid or soft fats, properly described as unsaturated, are found in vegetable oils, soft margarines and certain foods, including nuts and oily fish. Saturated fats are found in meat and meat products as well as in milk, butter, cream and cheese.

Much has been made of the so-called Mediterranean diet and its health-giving properties. This is a generic term referring to a diet that is rich in cardio-protective foods, which is certainly not the diet of the typical Briton. The Mediterranean diet contains large quantities of fresh fruit and vegetables, cereals, oily fish, pulses and olive oil. It is beneficial for many reasons, but particularly because it helps prevent weight gain, reduces cholesterol levels and in many cases helps protect against chronic heart disease.

If you prefer not to switch completely to this sort of diet, you should nevertheless:

- Aim for a diet low in saturated fatty acids by selecting reduced fat milk and dairy products, as well as going easy on red meat, cakes and pastries.
- Increase your intake of oily fish and unsaturated fatty acids.
- Increase the amount of soluble fibre in your diet such as is found in vegetables, fruit and high-fibre breads. These foods tend to be filling without being fattening, and some types of fibre, such as those found in oats and pulses, can help reduce blood cholesterol levels. Weight management

is also helped here because fibre promotes a feeling of fullness, so the temptation to eat more is reduced.

● Increase the amount of soya protein in your diet. There is now good evidence that soya-based protein can reduce harmful LDL cholesterol levels in the blood.

● Keep salt off the table. Don't add it to cooking either, as there is no question that we are all eating much more salt in our diet than we were 100 years ago. An increased salt intake pushes up our blood pressure and one clever Australian study showed that if workers who put salt on their food cut down on this (by reducing the number of holes in their salt shakers), their blood pressure fell significantly over an eight-week period.

● Eat at least five portions of fruit and vegetables a day. This is one of the best-known dietary principles at present and has been heavily promoted by the British Dietetic Association. Eating fresh fruit and vegetables has proven health benefits, because of their high content of antioxidants, which protect blood vessels from damage caused by the by-products of the body's cell metabolism. Examples of antioxidants are vitamins C and E and beta-carotene.

There are also well-recognised ways of assisting weight loss without the trauma of hunger pangs driving you to the nearest chip shop. My preferred ones include:

● Eat breakfast like a king, lunch like a lord and supper like a pauper. A hearty, low-fat breakfast reduces the likelihood of mid-morning snacking, as well as promoting concentration and energy until midday.

- Never crash-diet. Losing one or two pounds a week is absolutely fine.
- Eat slowly, savouring your food. This not only promotes enjoyment of food but also allows you to feel full before pudding arrives.
- Keep to a low-fat diet but don't cut out fats totally as your body needs them to function normally.
- Eat smaller meals more often and avoid late-night meals or snacks. Try using a smaller plate – you might be surprised at how effective this is.
- Use oil-free salad dressings, low-fat spreads, fat-free yoghurts and fresh fruit as often as possible. Trim fat off meat and don't eat the skin of poultry.

KEY POINTS

- Obesity is the second biggest cause, after smoking, of preventable disease in the developed world.
- Getting fat after 50 is not inevitable.
- Diet should always be part of a healthy lifestyle that should also include exercise, rest, laughter and variety.
- Avoid fad diets or crash diets – they never work.
- Above all, keep it simple.

OVER-50S MEN'S HEALTH CHECKLIST

- Know what your ideal weight should be, try to reach it and stick to it
- Eat a well-balanced diet rich in fresh fruit and vegetables
- Don't add salt to food during cooking or at table
- Keep consumption of sugar and fat to a minimum
- Drink eight glasses of water every day
- Keep consumption of alcohol to no more than 21 units a week
- Do everything you can to stop smoking
- Have your cholesterol level checked
- Have your blood pressure checked
- Have your PSA (prostate specific antigen) level checked
- Exercise regularly, even if it is just a brisk walk several times a week
- Engage in a wide variety of activities to keep both mind and body in trim
- Report any health concerns to your doctor
- Take all medication as prescribed, and report any serious side effects to your doctor

INDEX